MEDICAL CARE REFORM
A Guide to Issues and Choices

by
Henry A. Shenkin, M.D.

Oakvale Press
2431 32nd Street
Santa Monica, CA 90405

ISBN 0-9638888-4-6

LCCN 93-86677

ATTENTION HEALTH CARE GROUPS, ORGANIZATIONS, CORPORATIONS, AND EDUCATIONAL INSTITUTIONS: Quantity discounts are available on bulk purchases of this book for educational purposes or fund raising. Special books or book excerpts can also be created to fit specific needs. For information, please contact Oakvale Press, 2431 32nd Street, Santa Monica, California 90405, or call (310) 452-2769.

CONTENTS

iv

Preface

When I was a child growing up on Pine Street in Philadelphia, I got special attention in the neighborhood. People took my hand to cross the street, so I wouldn't get hit by a car - or a horse. They did this, they'd say, because I was *their doctor's* son. It was an era when people still revered their doctors. My father, who began practicing in 1900, belonged to a generation of physicians who could do very little for their patients medically - they didn't even have antibiotics - yet who were very well-respected. When I began to treat patients in 1939, I still felt this reverence for the doctor. But a decade or two later I began gradually to feel some measure of disrespect, even at times hostility, toward the profession, if not toward myself personally. How ironic that this breakdown of the doctor-patient relationship has occurred in an era when doctors help patients in ways that past generations would have called miraculous.

But when I retired in 1982, after 40 years of practicing neurosurgery, practice was not excruciatingly different from the one my father left when he died in 1933. A recent experience, however, showed me how drastically the profession has changed in the last decade. Contacting my former residents for a reunion, I made a surprising discovery: on the one hand, they feel frustrated by bureaucratic interference in their practices. On the other hand, they have earned far more money than I did before retiring 11 years ago. Thus, many of my former residents told me they plan to retire as soon as they turn 55.

These are personal experiences that tell me that something is drastically wrong with our current system of medical-care delivery in the United States. But the experience of many other Americans, unfortunately, leads them to agree. We all know that the price of medical care is skyrocketing, that the number of those unable to afford health insurance is rising, and that doctors are disgusted and discouraged by the endless paperwork and the hassle in their medical practices. Our system, although it still leads the world with its therapeutic innovations and quality of care for those who can afford it, has begun to plague us. It is a constant source of public dissatisfaction, and a financial weight which threatens to drag down our entire economy. As a political issue, it has determined the outcome of more than one election, and is likely to take an ever more prominent role in our country's political future.

While many people have made proposals for solving our medical-care crisis, I've also found that the problems are so complex that even the most informed of my doctor friends are not fully aware of the evolution of events in medical care. Other friends and acquaintances, although often very interested in the problem, haven't been able to learn systematically about the details and facts of the crisis and the proposed solutions. Article after article has appeared in newspapers and magazines, and many radio talk and television discussion shows have dealt with our medical-care problems. But the complexity of the crisis is such that most people can't even understand the terminology needed to describe it.

Thus I decided to write this guide.

Past experiences and reflections have already led to my writing two books. *Clinical Practice and Cost Containment* published by Praeger in 1986, analyzes the Canadian and British medical-care delivery systems, advocating emulation of the latter in the United States. *Medical Ethics: Evolution, Rights and the Physician* published by Kluwer in 1991, describes the causes of and the ethical problems arising from the deterioration of the doctor-patient relationship in this country.

But while this present book looks at the factors leading to the medical-care crisis and surveys the proposals to resolve it, it doesn't support any particular remedy or offer a program. It is simply meant to help anyone wishing for a comprehensive understanding of medical-care reform issues in order to form an intelligent opinion.

The data and material for this guide to issues and choices originated from references given in my book *Clinical Practice and Cost Containment*. This factual basis has been expanded over the last three years by collating and organizing additional material culled from a variety of professional journals and news sources. During that time I also collected data from governmental agency reports and various research organizations. The journals I consulted include *Journal of the American Medical Association, New England Journal of Medicine, Lancet, British Medical Journal, Bulletin of American College of Surgeons, Annals of Internal Medicine,* and *Science.* News sources included *The New York Times, Wall Street Journal, Philadelphia Inquirer, The Economist, U.S. News and World Report, American Medical News,* the *AARP Bulletin,* and *Update,* a publication of the National Academy of Social Insurance.

Introduction

The medical-care delivery system of the United States is in crisis.

Two Factors Shape the Medical-care Crisis

Two factors shape the national debate on the medical-care crisis: a meteoric rise in the cost of medical care, and the fact that a significant proportion of our population at any given time - in 1991, 36.3 million or 16.6% of Americans under 65 - has no access to it. Past actions to broaden access have always worsened cost escalation, because there were no accompanying incentives to providers or patients to economize on care. It's this direct relationship between access and costs that continues to plague efforts to solve the medical-care crisis in the United States.

It is important to distinguish between medical care and health care. Medical care consists of diagnosing and treating disease, and is only one aspect of health care which also comprehends preventive care and socio-economic factors impinging on people's health. When the crisis in health care in the U.S. is mentioned, it is almost exclusively the medical-care aspect that is meant. Perversely, many of the statistics cited - infant and maternal mortality, incidence of low-birth-weight babies and longevity - as evidence of medical care, are more reflective of the other aspects of health care.

Who Shall Be Insured?

Most Americans see universal access to medical care as a basic individual right, and therefore a matter of social justice. Universal access also contributes to the welfare and success of the nation, since it promotes the efficiency of its work force. Though there is considerable evidence that health is related markedly more to socio-economic status than access to medical care, most Americans believe that poverty should not be a barrier to universal access: through insurance or taxation, they believe costs of medical care should be spread among all the people. Agreement on this last principle has meant that Americans who don't have insurance or can't afford to pay out-of-pocket nevertheless receive some medical care, the costs of which almost always are "shifted" - paid for by increases in private insurance premiums.

Even though most American businesses have been spending more and more for their employees' health insurance, at any given time in 1991 there were still 26 million workers without insurance. Their numbers continue to grow steadily. Surprisingly, most of the uninsured are employed - in 1991, about 78% worked at least 18 hours a week - or were dependents of someone employed, usually by a small business. Even though mostly employed, the uninsured are predominantly poor: in 1992, 38.8% were in families with incomes below the federal poverty level ($14,343 for a family of four), and two-thirds in families with incomes below twice the poverty level. Medicaid (federal health program for the poor) varies from state to state, but overall it covered only 46% of those below the poverty level in 1988 despite its being the fastest accelerating state expenditure. Moreover, Medicaid reimburses at a rate far below private insurers or Medicare, so that many providers avoid caring for Medicaid patients.

How Much Care

Even though Americans may agree on universal access to health care, the question still remains: "How much health care are we talking about?" Most U.S. planners envision expanding benefits to include the basic elements of care: physician and hospital services (especially, care for pregnant women and children); prescription drugs; and long-term care (LTC) for permanently disabled people, particularly the aged. (Although the American system doesn't currently provide funding for LTC and drugs, most medical-care systems abroad do.) Most planners recognize the need to limit insured care - perhaps excluding, for example, psychiatric counseling and dentistry - but the amount of care included in many proposed programs is still beyond that now provided to most insured Americans.

Thus the need, both to universalize care and make it adequate add greatly to the projected costs of all the proposed programs. And the controversies among planners, physicians and politicians over the various programs revolves about what constitutes adequate care, and which benefits can be afforded. But if we are to overcome the medical-care crisis, such costs have to be offset by cost control measures.

Rising Costs of Medical Care

The cost of health care in the U.S. by 1991 had reached $738 billion or 13.2% of the gross domestic product (GDP). These costs reached $838.5 billion in 1992. Hospitals accounted for 38% of costs, doctors 19%, drugs 8%, supplies 15% and administration 20%. In 1992, costs were accelerating 12% per year, outstripping all other items in the cost-of-living index, and between 1992 and 2000 health care costs were projected to rise from $2700 per individual to $5100 (projected to be 18.1% of GDP in the year 2000). Medical care costs accounted for 14% of the average American family's spending in 1991, as compared with 5% and 8% in Britain and Canada, respectively. The costs are so high that American families who make less than $20,000-a-year worry more about health costs than about finding a job or paying the rent.

Yet despite this high expenditure on health care, many U.S. health statistics are cited as lagging behind other advanced nations. For instance, American women with an average life expectancy of 78.6 years in 1991 were in 16th place internationally. American men, with an average life span of 71.6 years, tended to die sooner than men in 22 other countries. The U.S. lags behind Western Europe in infant mortality; behind Greece, Italy and Spain in maternal mortality; and behind Jordan, Ireland and Costa Rica in the incidence of low-birth-weight babies. Children in Greece and Czechoslovakia are more likely to be vaccinated against polio than children in the United States. One might say that the above statistics by themselves don't prove medical care abroad is equal or better for all than in the United States. And available data indicates that, for the many Americans who can afford care, their length and quality of life are better here than elsewhere. However, many societies abroad are satisfied with their medical-care systems. And that is indisputedly not so in the United States.

There is a great deal of concern, too, that our country's huge medical-care expenditures are eroding its competitive position with other advanced nations, since employers pay out the bulk of this money. While the U.S. in 1989 spent 11.8% of its GDP on health care Japan spent 6.7%, Germany 8.2%, Britain 5.9%, Canada 8.7%, Sweden 8.8%, Holland 8.3% and France 8.7%. In other terms, the U.S. spent $2,354 on health care per person that year, to be compared with $1,035 by Japan, $1,232 by Germany, Britain's $836, Canada's $1,683, Sweden's $1,361, France's $1,274 and Italy's $1,050.

Finally, the excessive cost of health care is a major contributor to the exorbitant U.S. national debt. Federal spending on both Medicaid and Medicare is rising rapidly. Medicaid expenditures rose 28% in 1991 and 29% in 1992, to $67.8 billion. Medicare spending increased 7% in 1991 and 12% in 1992, to $116 billion. Thus the Congressional Budget Office has estimated that health care adds an extra 1% of GNP ($60 billion in 1991) to the budget deficit every year.

Why Do Medical-care Costs Keep Going Up?

The main cause of escalating medical-care costs over the past fifty years has been the increased access to medical care afforded by the expansion of private insurance plans (such as Blue Cross and Blue Shield), along with the introduction of government-sponsored and funded plans (Medicare and Medicaid). These expansions increased medical-care costs not only by expanding the number of people with access to care, but also by making care appear to be cost-free at the time of use. That appearance encouraged people to seek medical care more (insured people use at least 40% more care than similar uninsured persons). Not only did no essential changes in delivery of care accompany this expansion of access, but providers like hospitals and doctors had the economic incentive to dispense as much care as possible.

Why, when this expansion of access and demand occurred, were no steps taken to keep costs from skyrocketing? In order to convince hospitals, doctors and other providers to accept government medical-care programs, legislators agreed that Medicare and Medicaid would pay doctors their usual and customary fees and hospitals on a cost-plus basis. Private insurers generally followed the patterns of payments set by public payers.

Administrative expenses and the current tort system also contribute to the rising costs of medical care. High administrative costs, caused in great part by the complexity in the reporting and paying for services and insurance company profits, total $100 to $160 billion per year. The entire U.S. tort system used up $132 billion in 1991, including $5.6 billion for doctor and $9 billion for hospital malpractice insurance, and an estimated $15.1 billion for "defensive medicine". Both the administrative and litigative-climate costs of the U.S. medical-care system are not only greater than those in other nations but also, for purposes of future discussion, fall within the definition of "unnecessary medical care" (see Chapter II, Rationing).

Finally, there are two even more important causes of the acceleration in medical-care costs. These are the aging of the population, and new technology. Both of these create the need for more "necessary care" - medical care that prolongs life and/or contributes to its quality.

The aging of the population, as in all the advanced industrialized nations, increases the need for both acute and long-term care (LTC). In 1989, people over 65 accounted for 12% of the population (30 million) but used 36% of medical-care costs.

Approximately 3.9% of the population need LTC services, of whom 40% to 51% of these people are under 65 years of age. About 3.6% of the total non-institutionalized population need assistance with activities of daily living, including 8% of those aged 65 to 69, and 46% of those over 85. In 1990, 1.5 million people were in nursing homes and 200,000 were in psychiatric and long- stay hospitals at a total cost of about $50 billion.

Since the aged part of the population can't pay for all of this LTC, the burden reverts to the whole nation. Private insurance covers less than 1% of Americans' need for LTC, and then needed services are only partially covered. About half of LTC expenses are paid out-of-pocket and the rest, $35 billion, by Medicaid (for many, after having "spent down" their assets to qualify for Medicaid). The elderly spend 18% of their income for health care, with out-of-pocket expenses rising twice as fast as social security payments. Medicaid coverage spends far more on nursing homes than for home- and community-based services. The way Medicaid was structured deprives the young-poor of coverage: it covers only 42% of the individuals whose income falls below the federal poverty level despite Medicaid being the fastest growing expenditure for many states. Medicaid recipients grew by only 9% from 1980 to 1989, while costs rose 123% and the principal reason was that the long-term care provided the elderly in nursing homes (7% of all Medicaid recipients) took 50% of the Medicaid budget. Medicaid covers almost two thirds of the 1.5 million nursing home residents.

If financial barriers were removed, estimates are that demand for LTC would leap to about $90 billion a year. This would include a 20% increase in nursing home utilization, and a 50 to 100% increase in demand for community services for those at home (which cost $8 billion in 1990).

An explosion of new and expensive medical technology in this latter part of the 20th century has increased considerably the cost of medical care in all advanced nations, but especially in the United States where there is little means to control the supply and usage of such innovations. Insurers say that as much as 40% of their recent annual increases in premiums in recent years is due to the use of new technology.

Drug innovations have also contributed to the escalation in medical-care costs. Over the last decade their cost rose three times faster than general inflation (147% compared to 50%). The United States is the only advanced industrial nation without any mechanism to control the prices of drugs. As a result, the total cost of drugs in the United States will reach an estimated $72 billion in 1993.

However, the cost of drugs represent only 8% of the total health care costs in the United States in 1991. Americans spend far less on drugs per capita - $268 per year - than do their German or Japanese counterparts, who spent $526 and $390 respectively in 1991. This occurs even though Germany and Japan spend far less, overall, on medical care than does the United States.

To summarize then, the increased access to medical care afforded by creating and expanding private and government insurance plans, high administrative costs, the current tort system, the aging of the population and the availability of new technologies are combining to make the costs of health care in the United States skyrocket. At the same time, our dominant social and political philosophy holds that all

Americans should have access to medical care - a situation which inevitably raises costs as well.

The first chapter of this book expands on the causes of the crisis in the American medical-care system and reviews previous incremental efforts at reform. Although these attempts met with little success, it's important to review them in preparation for a look at the comprehensive reform programs now under consideration (Chapter V).

While "unnecessary care" costs such as administrative costs can, theoretically, be controlled by governmental regulation or legislation, control of the acceleration in costs of "necessary care" requires some form of rationing. Because of the importance of rationing to the issue of cost containment, the second chapter of this book is devoted to that subject.

Chapter III reviews in some detail medical-care systems of other industrialized nations. Some of these are being suggested as models for U.S. reform. We will see that many of the same factors escalating costs in the United States are affecting these other nations, which in turn are also instituting changes in their systems.

Chapter IV reviews the ideologic considerations underlying health reform efforts and summarizes the methods available for accomplishing reform. Chapter V classifies and summarizes the various programs being offered to reform the U.S. medical-care delivery system. Chapter VI presents the influence of the political realities of a representative democracy on any effort at medical-care reform.

Finally, following the final chapter, I have provided a glossary and list of acronyms to help readers glide as easily as possible through this most complicated subject.

Table Intro-1
Problems Leading to Crisis in Health Care

1. Lack of access:

   A. need for universal access

      (1)   it is a right
      (2)   a factor in welfare and success of nation (via health of work force)

   B. need for adequate care - long-term care as well as all phases of acute care

2. Acceleration of costs:

   A. effect on individual
   B. effect on nation

      (1)   competitive position of business
      (2)   contribution to nation's debt

Table Intro-2
Causes of Medical-care Cost Increases

1. Increasing "unnecessary care" (#)

   A. Insurance makes care appear of no cost to patient
   B. Cost-plus and fee-for-service payment to providers
   C. Malpractice litigation and defensive medicine
   D. Burgeoning administrative costs

2. Escalation of "necessary care" (*)

   A. Aging of population
   B. New technology

(# =rationing not required   * = rationing required)

Chapter I

Previous Attempts to Solve Problems in Delivery of Medical Care

Past Efforts to Expand Access

Health insurance is, of course, the most obvious way to expand access to medical care, since it reduces the cost to the individual by spreading it among many people - including some who won't use it at all. Insurance in the United States doesn't merely leave intact the entrepreneurial delivery of medical care, but in fact enhances providers' profits.

There are two kinds of insurance: experience-rated (casualty or risk-rated) and community-rated. Experience-rated insurance sets premiums according to the expected cost of claims by individual applicants based on the likelihood of their need for medical care in the reasonably foreseeable future. Thus, insurance premiums rates can be kept down by the exclusion of individuals based on their previous health status, age, sex, occupation, or geographic location. Insurers can also charge risky individuals much higher - often non-affordable - rates. Experience-rating insurers generally charge higher rates to small businesses than to larger groups, such as large corporations. That's because the high-risk individuals in a small group are more costly to an insurer than they would be when submerged in the greater numbers of a large organization.

Community-rated insurance premiums are uniform for all, regardless of individual or group risks. The rate is set by the exposure

1

to risk of the entire population. That means the young, healthy and single subsidize the elderly, those with pre-existing conditions and those with large families. The young also pay in advance for medical care they are likely to use when they're older.

Many people believe risk-rated premiums are fairer than the community-rated, especially to low risk individuals, since 5% of the population incur 50% of all health expenses, and only 10% of the population incur 70% of all such expenses. However, mandating that insurance companies use community-rating rather than experience-rating for premiums, increases access to medical care without serving to contain its costs. Indeed, by itself, universalizing community-rated premiums tends to increase expenditures on medical care, since it makes coverage affordable for more people. Moreover, since it raises premiums for the young and healthy, they are encouraged to forego insurance - defeating the very purpose of those advocating this approach.

Nevertheless, by 1992, 14 states had taken steps toward requiring health insurance companies to community-rate their premiums.

A second means of expanding access to medical care is for the state to pay all or part of the premiums for low-income people. This is the idea behind Medicaid. But the acceleration in Medicaid's cost to the states (even though the cost is shared, about equally, by the federal government) has led to increasing restrictions in its eligibility rules, reducing accessibility to care for many poor people. Nevertheless, most of the various proposed plans usually recommend that premiums be totally subsidized for people living at or below poverty level (in 1992, $13,400 for a family of four and $6620 for an individual), and partially subsidized for those with incomes between 100% and 200% of the poverty level.

Past Efforts at Cost Containment

Despite their inadequacy, past initiatives to control costs continue to be included in many of the proposed new plans. Indeed, many believe that the only option is more vigorous pursuit of such "incremental changes", since any overall reform of the system is not feasible politically.

Previous cost containment efforts principally targeted the overuse and expansion of hospitals, since hospitals costs used to account for

45% of the total cost of medical care. Since most hospitals had been built or enlarged with federal grants and since many derive a large portion of their revenue from Medicare and Medicaid, the effort to control their costs has largely been through congressional legislation or federal governmental regulation.

By 1992, hospital costs were down to 38% of the total costs of medical care, with 19% going to doctors, 23% for drugs and supplies and 20% for administration. Since the rate of escalation in doctors' pay has far exceeded both the in rise cost of living and the growth in GNP, the federal government is attempting to curb doctors' fees. The government is trying not only to contain the escalation in doctors' charges to Medicare, but also to equalize payments to the various types of physicians (see below under RBRVSs).

When Medicare has changed the way it pays medical-care providers, private insurers have usually followed suit. One can assume that whenever government regulates Medicare reimbursements for cost containment purposes, these changes will, sooner or later, apply to the private insurance payers as well.

Partial Payment of Premiums (Deductibles) and Co-Payments

Sometimes an employer or the government provides insurance for individuals, but requires the insured to pay part of the premium. This kind of "partial payment" steers people toward plans with the lowest premiums. Requiring the insured patient to pay a certain amount "out-of-pocket" before the insurance takes over payment for services is an even more efficient cost containment measure. Such partial out-of-pocket payments are known as deductibles. "Copayments" or "balance-of-payments" also require the insured patient to pay part of the fee for some or all services.

Exclusion of drugs from the benefits of many, if not most, U.S. insurance plans, including Medicare, contain costs similarly to deductibles and copayments. Individuals pay more than 50% of the cost of drugs and this percentage is growing; in 1992, retirees were paying more out-of-pocket for drugs than for medical or hospital care.

Copayments and deductibles reduce demand for office visits more than for hospitalizations. A study by the Rand Corporation showed that families required to absorb the first $1000 a year of their medical costs spent 40% less than those with no insurance deductibles. One would hope that people with deductibles avoid only unnecessary medical treatment, but this is not likely. Nor do deductibles eliminate all unnecessary care. Indeed, these methods of inhibiting the use of insurance for medical care are really marketplace rationing methods: the more affluent are not inhibited at all, and the less affluent are inhibited too much. Deductibles and copayments, while restraining costs, dilute the goal of increasing access to medical care.

Peer Review

In 1972 Congress established Professional Standards Review Organizations (PSROs) in an attempt to control Medicare and Medicaid expenditures. The legislation was based on two concepts: first, that physicians are the most appropriate individuals to assess the quality of patient care; and second, that local peer review is the best way to ensure appropriate use of federally financed (i.e., through Medicare and Medicaid) medical-care resources and facilities.

The 1972 amendment to the Social Security Act mandated that committees of hospital staff physicians review their own hospital's admissions and lengths of stay. Local (city, county, or similar areas) PSRO established standards that were applied to all hospitals in their area. The hospital committee determined the appropriateness and estimated the length of stay of all admissions shortly after the patient entered the hospital. Any stay that exceeded the estimate was subsequently reviewed. If the hospital's own reviewers found the hospital admission or length of stay unjustified, they recommended denying reimbursement to the hospital for that admission or excessive stay. If a hospital did not conform to local standards for hospital utilization or review process, the PSRO organization of that locality assigned outside reviewers.

But the PSRO program didn't stem the progressive rise in hospital costs. So Congress in 1982 passed the Tax Equity and Fiscal Responsibility Act (TEFRA), which repealed the old PSRO system and established a new Utilization and Quality Control Peer Review Organization system. TEFRA reduced the number of peer review groups by making their oversight areas statewide or regional, rather than local. It also allowed payer groups, such as insurers, to serve as review panels if no physician groups were available. But organized medicine did not resist PSROs, and the vast majority of PSRO contracts went to physician groups.

The new review groups based their judgments on a prospective payment system relying on diagnosis-related groups (DRGs, see below). Their purpose is to prevent doctors and hospitals from circumventing the latter by: increasing the number of hospital admissions; by premature discharge of patients and re-admission thereafter; by transferring patients to psychiatric or rehabilitative units (which were exempt from DRG rates); admitting patients with multiple problems several times instead of treating all problems at the same time; or admitting patients for procedures that could be done as outpatients. Even though the review groups are called Physicians' or Peer Review Organizations they are in fact staffed not by doctors but by lower paid personnel such as registered or experienced practical nurses or "audit retrieval technicians".

Second Opinion Programs

A second opinion program is a peer review procedure specifically designed to reduce elective surgeries. It requires that a second surgeon agree to the necessity, or to the desirability, of a non-emergency operation before the insurance company or HMO agrees to pay for it. Private insurers and HMOs have demanded second opinions, but the federal government never has. Results of cost-effectiveness studies of second opinion programs conflict. But it is clear that any savings reaped by such program have not been significant. The studies found that the second opinion most often agreed with the first or, when they conflicted, the patient frequently wanted the procedure.

Certificate-of-Need Program (CON)

This program was designed to control capital expansion of hospitals. It required governmental agency approval for sizable capital expenditures, and issuance of a certificate-of-need before adding to or altering a hospital, or before acquiring proposed equipment. States administered the program according to guidelines issued by the U.S. Department of Health and Human Services. The guidelines were designed to prevent costly excess capacity and duplication of services.

Originally under the Certificate-of-Need program a hospital wishing to make a capital expenditure of more than $100,000 had to obtain a CON. In 1985 the threshold was raised to $275,000 for any new equipment, $400,000 for any medical technology system, and $680,000 for renovations. Federally-funded local committees of the state Health Systems Agency decided whether to grant the CON, and the decisions were then reviewed by the state Secretary of Health. However, over the years, this program has had little effect on hospital expenditures. Nor did it reduce hospitals' dollar investments because local political pressures helped hospitals to circumvent most CON requirements.

Prospective Payment System (PPS) According to Diagnostic Related Groups (DRGs)

This program was phased in from 1983 to 1986. It aims to control Medicare hospital costs, which had grown from $3 billion per year in 1967 to $140 billion in 1993. By that same year, Medicare and Medicaid payments combined represented about 45% of an average hospital's revenue. Medicare, like Blue Cross and other insurance companies, had previously reimbursed hospitals for "reasonable costs" incurred in caring for a patient, with no set limits. Congress mandated the DRG system when it became obvious that neither hospitals nor doctors would contain costs voluntarily.

The DRG system classifies patients into 467 groups. Groups are determined according to diagnosis on admission to the hospital; age and sex; whether the treatment is medical or surgical; whether there are secondary diagnoses; and discharge destination. Then the hospital's reimbursement rate is determined by a complex methodology which includes factors such as hospital location (urban or rural); local wage rates (since labor represents 70% of hospital costs); and a "case mix index" - which essentially classifies a hospital as community, acute-care, tertiary referral, or related to a medical school or medical center. The remuneration rate is also affected by the region of the country in which the hospital is located. Two types of atypical patients are allowed additional payments: "day outliers" who stay in hospitals extremely long lengths of time; and "cost outliers" who involve extraordinary costs. Although they bring in extra payments, outliers represent a great loss to a hospital. Hospital outpatient services, certain types of hospitals, and certain distinct units within hospitals (psychiatric, long-term care, pediatrics and rehabilitation) are exempt from the Medicare DRG prospective payment system.

The essence of the DRG prospective payment system is that hospitals receive a flat fee for a diagnostic category no matter what the cost to the hospital. Thus, the shorter the stay and the fewer the diagnostic tests and other services a patient receives, the more the hospital will profit from the admission.

Since private insurers usually follow federal program reimbursement patterns, they too adopted the DRG program.

The immediate impact of the DRG prospective payment system was that hospital administrations encouraged and pressured their doctors to reduce the number of laboratory and diagnostic tests ordered on patients, and to reduce patients' stay in the hospital. These pressures aren't detrimental to most patients, but they can be harmful to patients sicker than the average of their DRG. The system also encourages early discharge of patients, often placing a burden on their families.

Thus "DRG creep" has developed: doctors tend to put patients' diagnoses in less accurate but better-remunerated categories. The DRG system has also produced a tendency for hospitals to "unbundle" their services. Unbundling means separating out and billing by ostensibly independent physicians for services previously supplied by a hospital, such as x-rays or anesthesia. Part B of Medicare (physician reimbursement) rather than Part A (hospital reimbursement) then pays the bill. DRG creep and unbundling, as well as more active "cost-shifting" and political pressures to prevent some hospital failures have combined to prevent the DRG prospective payment system from completely controlling the inordinate inflation of hospital costs in the United States.

Resource-Based Relative Value Scale for Physicians' Reimbursement (RBRVSs)

This program was mandated for Medicare payments to doctors by Congress in 1989, and went into effect January 1, 1992. The law intended to reduce overall payments to doctors by 6% (after inflation); and to adjust payments in a way that would de-emphasize specialty charges, especially for "procedures", and increase the compensation for "cognitive activity", i.e., knowing or thinking. This program also aims to increase fees to primary physicians and decrease those to specialists. Thus payments to radiologists, pathologists, anesthesiologists and surgeons decreased, while those for general practitioners, generalists and internists increased.

While RBRVSs do attempt to make physician fees more equitable, their primary aim is to reduce medical-care costs. Thus, to ensure that physicians don't increase their services to compensate for any curtailment of their fees under RBRVSs, Congress also established Medicare Volume Performance Standards (MVPSs). MVPSs set annual targets for expenditures under the Medicare Part B. If expenditures in any year exceed the target, fee adjustments are to be made in the following year. That means if expenditures are higher than the MVPS target one year, fees will be decreased the next year, and increased if expenditures are lower than the target.

Under RBRVSs, fees are based on the relative values established for three service components: 1) a work component unit reflecting the physician's time and intensity; 2) a practice expense unit component that reflects overhead; and 3) a malpractice component unit reflecting malpractice costs. While the relative value units assigned to each component of a particular service are the same throughout the country, the absolute value of each component is adjusted to reflect geographic variations. The fee is the same for a specific service whether or not the physician is a specialist. By the summer of 1991, fee schedules had been established for more than 4500 physicians' services. This new payment schedule is to be phased in over 5 years, through 1996.

RBRVSs have been criticized because their charge-based components (overhead and malpractice-cost portions) are set at 46% and the resource-based (work) component at 56%. Critics say that the charge-based component is set too high to make physicians' clinical decisions financially neutral. On the other hand, many say that the annual setting of the rate conversion factor at the discretion of government without prescribed guidelines will surely result in under-compensation of doctors. That is because budgetary pressures are likely to outweigh all other considerations in setting the rate of increase in physicians' fees under Medicare, and consequently by all third-party payment plans. The critics point out that RBRVSs don't address the true causes of increased spending on physicians' services.

These causes are the rising number of physicians, the constantly increasing new technologies and new uses for old ones, and the extensive use of gap insurance (supplementary or secondary insurance) for Medicare deductibles and copayments). The continued rise in patients' expectations and the incentives built into the fee-for-service system of compensation also contribute to the increased spending.

Health Maintenance Organizations (HMOs), including Individual Practice Associations (IPAs)

HMOs, which began in 1971 under the Nixon administration, have grown slowly, but steadily. In recent years they have grown 4-5% annually, and by 1992 covered 37 million people including 23% of employed families. HMOs heaviest enrollments are in large cities, especially in the far and middle west. In 1992 49% of the population of San Francisco belonged to HMOs, 46% in Minneapolis and between 32 and 35% in Milwaukee, Portland and Los Angeles. Between 22 and 28% of the population in Boston, Denver, Phoenix, Seattle and Washington, D.C. belonged to HMOs. Most of this expansion has occurred in the IPA form of HMOs (see below).

In their purest form, HMOs enroll subscribers who pay a single fee up front, to cover all their medical needs, including doctor visits, diagnostic studies, and hospitalization. The HMO employs physicians, and often contracts with or own hospitals. These kinds of HMOs are known as staff-type or group-model HMOs. In 1992, there were 15 million subscribers to this kind of HMO. Staff-model HMOs employ doctors and, by now, most have been set up by an entrepreneurial organization (for-profit HMO). In the group-model, the physicians are an independent aggregate that provides its services, exclusively, to the HMO, which is, generally, non-profit.

The theory behind HMOs is the same as for all prospective payment systems: to give providers a financial incentive to economize on services. The fewer tests done and hospitalizations recommended, the larger the portion of the pool of pre-paid fees that will be available to be divided among the physicians of a "non-profit" HMO, or go to the owners of a "for-profit" HMO. Since doctors control these services, they have the incentive to minimize them. Also, the fewer surgical and other specialty consultations, the greater the income of the primary physician (often referred to as a "managing physician") in an HMO.

Theoretically, professional ethics prevent HMO physicians from denying their patients necessary care. However, critics say that HMOs impair professional ethics, since patients don't choose physicians, who in turn don't provide "continuity of care". These are two circumstances that ordinarily "bind" doctors and patients. Many HMOs do permit patients to choose among their member doctors and do provide some measure of continuity of care. However, many doctors are attracted to HMOs for the regular hours and vacations they provide, which in turn inhibit continuity of care.

While initially HMOs were non-profit, for-profit organizations eventually entered the field. By 1992 an estimated two thirds of HMOs were investor owned. Commercial and Blue-Cross insurers have successfully marketed their own HMOs; there are at least seven other HMO companies with publicly traded stock. While for-profit HMOs have the same incentive as the non-profits to limit unnecessary care, their owners are not constrained by any professional ethic. Critics accuse them of imposing on their employee physicians unrealistic standards for the number of tests, consultations and hospitalizations they recommend, or authorize at the request of patients.

HMOs also come in the form of groupings of physicians called individual practice associations or IPAs. IPA physicians maintain their own offices and care for subscribers to one or more prepaid plans on a fee-for-service basis, at a negotiated reduction of rates. Also called "network type HMOs" or "point-of-service plans", these kinds of organizations had 24,000,000 subscribers in 1992, making them the largest form of HMO.

IPAs have not been as cost-effective as the staff- or group- type HMOs, because IPA physicians are paid more when they perform more services, and therefore have less incentive to curtail services. Studies have found staff-type HMOs' medical-care cost is 17% lower per employee than traditional health insurance plans and 8% lower for IPAs.

While HMOs have since their inception lowered expenditures, the rate of acceleration in their costs have matched that of the other medical-care sectors.

The growth of HMOs and their dependence on primary physicians to "manage care" has exposed the severe shortage of general practitioners in the United States. This shortage has occurred because third-party payment policies have increased the earning power of specialists so much more than primary physicians. In addition, governmental policy through Medicare and Medicaid gives teaching hospitals extra payments (totaling $5.5 billion annually) to train residents as specialists. Both of these policies conspire to reduce society's regard for generalists as compared to specialists.

Preferred Provider Organizations (PPOs) or Preferred Provider Insurance (PPI)

PPOs are groups of hospitals and physicians offering fee-for-service care at reduced rates in return for a guaranteed volume of patients. Usually PPOs are organized by a hospital or hospitals and their staffs, or by an administrator who recruits physicians and hospitals for such a plan.

PPOs also claim to promote cost containment by providing utilization review, including pre-admission and pre-procedure certification, concurrent review of hospital stays, second surgical opinion programs, review of outpatient care, retrospective reviews and analysis of physicians' practice patterns (physician profiling). PPO consumers are most often companies, especially the self-insured, looking for ways to contain their employees medical benefits costs. Negotiated fee schedules are usually five to 20% less than the usual charges for services. Most often, PPOs are a reaction to a competitive threat perceived by the providers - for instance, the development of HMOs. Most PPOs have arisen in the far west, where prepaid plans are the strongest.

Since companies tended more to offer incentives to their employees for an HMO option than for a PPO, by 1991 only 17% of employed families belonged to PPOs as opposed to 23% using HMOs (55% continuing on a traditional fee-for-service basis). In 1991, the average cost per employer for a PPO was $3355, $3046 for an HMO and $3573 in the traditional fee-for-service setting.

While PPOs are also fee-for-service plans, the need to keep their costs competitive with HMOs and below that of prevalent insurance plans motivates their sponsors and physicians to use consultations and facilities judiciously. PPOs are thus categorized, on occasion, as a type of managed care. Patient participation in a PPO is never mandated by an employer. However, employees have an incentive to use the PPO because coverage for using other services is only at 80%. Although insurers stress that PPOs provide patients freedom-of-choice, the patients in fact have a strong financial incentive to select only PPO providers.

Since companies tend to offer employees stronger incentives to join HMOs rather than PPOs, by 1991 only 17% of employed families belonged to PPOs, while 23% used HMOs. Fifty-five percent of families continued with traditional fee-for-service plans. In 1991, the average cost per employee for a PPO was $3355, $3046 for an HMO and $3573 in the traditional fee-for-service setting.

Competitive Medical Organizations (CMOs)

CMOs are outgrowths of successful HMOs. They are voluntary, vertically integrated, regionally based, non-profit or for- profit, managed-care health delivery systems whose providers collaborate to provide comprehensive medical services. The key component of a CMO is a primary care focused multi-specialty group which may contract with affiliated independent physicians. Community hospitals, sometimes owned by the CMO, provide secondary care. Smaller, regional tertiary hospitals provide high technology services.

In addition, CMOs offer strategic planning, total quality management and management information systems, credentialing of physicians, utilization review and marketing services. Examples of developing CMOs are the Kaiser Foundation, Intermountain Health Care and Sutter Health, all in the Western United States.

Primary Care Networks

Primary Care Networks have been introduced principally for Medicaid patients. Funded by the states in combination with the federal government (50% to 70%), and administered by the states, Medicaid has been a particular object of regulation. When Medicaid began, freedom to choose one's provider was somewhat reduced; the Reagan administration wished to eliminate it entirely. Congress agreed to allow the states to arrange to purchase laboratory or medical services through competitive bids, to implement "managed primary care" systems (i.e. HMOs), and to allow assistance to recipients in selecting a provider from competing health plans. States are also permitted to establish a "lock-in" feature, which restricts choice of a provider by a beneficiary who has over-used services, as well as a "lock-out" feature, which limits the participation of particular "over-zealous" providers of Medicaid.

However, Congress required states to make contracts with only federally approved HMOs, because of some mishaps in California. That state had worked with several unapproved prepaid plans, which first used allegedly questionable and high-pressure techniques to enroll many Medicaid patients, then under-served them. This occurred even though the administration of the then-Governor Reagan had encouraged Medicaid of California to contract only with approved HMOs or "primary care networks".

A primary care network - also known as "case-managed care" - places primary care physicians at economic risk in order to make them use medical resources for their patients more prudently. Primary care networks consist of primary physicians and a panel of specialists. The primary physician must approve all referrals to the specialists. The primary physicians are paid in advance per capita for each patient. If they make excessive referrals or use of hospitals, their income is reduced. In some networks, participating specialists and hospitals are similarly at financial risk. In others, specialists and hospitals are paid on a fee-for-service basis at reduced rates, and hope to make up their fees by increased referrals.

Most primary care networks currently depend on Medicaid patients as their principal market, and favor patients receiving Aid-to-Families-with-Dependent-Children because they are the youngest and least costly to treat. (Although patients receiving AFDC constitute 63% of all Medicaid recipients, they represent only 28% of Medicaid expenditures).

Despite its objective, Medicaid still fails to provide health care to an estimated 60% of the poor. This is because many states restrict Medicaid to artificially low standards of income, typically one-fourth to one-third lower than the national poverty standard. Medicaid also typically allows applicants to hold no more than $1000 to $1500 in assets.

Although Medicare was the program designed to provide health care to the elderly, actually 29% of all Medicaid patients are aged, and they received 70% of Medicaid funds. A large portion of this amount goes toward long-term care in a nursing home for disabled (mostly old) people who have "spent-down" their assets. Seven percent of Medicaid patients spend 40% of Medicaid funds on nursing-home care.

Managed Care

Managed care most often refers to the group or staff model HMO concept (see above, under HMOs). This type of managed care gives providers an economic incentive to avoid excessive and unnecessary care.

However, managed care as provided in PPO or net-work type HMO is different, because it implies supervision of providers to prevent unnecessary or excessive care. Under this kind of managed-care system, patients either are assigned to a primary physician, or choose one from a panel recruited by the insurer into a network type HMO or PPO.

Most doctors prefer traditional fee-for-service practice because they retain their autonomy to act in the best interests of their patients. However, insurance companies (including Blue Cross and Blue Shield) control so many patients, especially in certain areas, that doctors feel compelled to accept reduced fees in order to maintain or expand their volume of practice. Managed care plans give insurance companies (or another payer) the power to force physicians to conform to their rules against "wasteful and unnecessary practices" or risk losing a steady source of patients and income. Insurance companies and other payers also use "physician profiling" to eliminate the care that is unnecessary, from their point of view. Physician profiling abroad is only for the prescribing of drugs.

Under this kind of managed care, not only do doctors receive reduced fees but all studies and treatments must initiate with, or be approved by, the managing doctor. If a patient requests a service on his own, or on the initiative of another doctor, the insurer will not pay for it without prior agreement by the managing doctor.

Most medical-care insurers have recently adopted a more punitive variation on supervised managed care. Before agreeing to pay, they insist on reviewing certain designated treatments and diagnostic studies ordered by doctors in traditional fee-for-service practice. The avowed objective of this stratagem is to contain costs by eliminating unnecessary services. However, doctors complain they are spending hours every day defending their own judgment against second-guessing by insurance company nurses and doctors, who have never seen their patients and sometimes have little knowledge of their specialties.

To sum up, the objections to managed care are that it gives physicians incentives which spills over to denying or delaying beneficial care, and that administrators sooner or later start determining care according to affordability under their plans. In addition, even if managed care is well run, the cost of collecting reliable data on the efficacy of various treatment, and the capital costs of developing managed-care networks offset any savings. Finally, after a decade of development, managed-care systems have not made a dent in the rate of escalation of medical-care costs. The reason may be that while managed care is designed to eliminate unnecessary care, aging and new technology are increasing the amount of necessary care.

Table I-1
Previous Incremental Attempts to Expand Access

1. Expansion of private insurance (Blue Cross, etc.)
2. Introduction of government insurance (Medicare, Medicaid)
3. Community rating of insurance premiums
4. Employer health insurance mandated by individual states

Table I-2
Previous Incremental Attempts at Cost-containment

1. Deductibles and copayments (including the cost of drugs)
2. Peer review (PSROs)
3. Second opinion programs
4. Certificate-of-need programs (CON)
5. Prospective payments according to diagnostic related groups (DRGs)
6. Resource-based relative value scale for physician reimbursements (RBRVSs)

7. Managed care

   A. health maintenance organizations (HMOs) & individual practice associations (IPAs)
   B. primary care networks
   C. preferred provider organizations (PPOs)
   D. direct supervision by insurers

8. Competitive medical organizations (CMOs)

Chapter II

Rationing

Medical care is rationed in every nation, by one means or another. Since it demands denying some care to some people, rationing has acquired a pejorative connotation. Therefore, rationing is seldom mentioned when discussing programs for reforming a medical-care system; planners believe that any mention of rationing will ruin chances of enacting a given reform plan.

But because all current health systems entail some form of rationing, it must be a necessity for curbing costs, or at least the easiest way to constrain them. Even the United States, the wealthiest of nations, rations health care, by limiting access to those that can't afford it.

Rationing is probably only needed for care that is "necessary" - care that prolongs life, or maintains or improves its quality - and not for "unnecessary care" which serves neither purpose. Acceleration in costs due to "unnecessary care" can likely be checked by means other than rationing.

Everyone agrees that free access to a medical-care delivery system encourages overuse of services. Giving doctors financial incentives to offer as many services as possible, as we do in the United States, aggravates that overuse. But the resulting "unnecessary care" can be controlled by regulations or legislation that change incentives for both patients and providers. Making patients pay out-of-pocket for at least part of the services they receive, and introducing prospective payments for doctors (as in managed care) are example of such regulations. Tort reform, too, would lessen physicians' fear of malpractice and the

17

resultant unnecessary testing and procedures of defensive medical practice.

On the other hand, aging of the population and the constant introduction of new and usually expensive technology are accelerating both the need for and costs of necessary medical care. But it's unlikely that the same measures that can reduce unnecessary care could acceptably or efficiently keep costs from spiraling due to necessary care. Reducing unnecessary care diminishes overall costs but, ultimately, only lowers the set-point from which cost acceleration caused by necessary care takes off. Hence it's the ability to ration necessary care that, in one way or another, has allowed advanced nations other than the United States to keep their health costs from rapidly accelerating over the past decade.

More recently, however, even the foreign systems are finding it increasingly difficult to control expenditures due to aging of *their* populations and the increase in new technologies.

There are several distinct methods of rationing. First, there are macro- or micro-rationing procedures. Macro-rationing occurs when government limits the total funds allocated to medical care, either through global budgeting, or through a single-payer mechanism for negotiation with providers and which can also simplify administration. (some governments use both methods.) These macro-rationing decisions, subsequently, are carried out by micro-rationing, that is, by deciding who shall have access to a specific procedure, the supply of which is constrained by the amount of funds allocated to medical care.

The proponents of global budgeting and/or single-payer methods for the United States well might believe that any constraints they impose on funding can be met by reducing costs and profits on health services and eliminating unnecessary utilization and thus avoid micro-rationing. But all such macro-rationing decisions abroad have been accompanied by the micro-rationing of necessary care.

Second, rationing can be implicit or explicit. It's implicit when decisions about who gets which care is not legally mandated but, nevertheless, generated by the nature of the delivery system. Implicit rationing is micro-rationing that is achieved either according to the patient's ability to pay, or by individual physicians making decisions on a case by case basis. It is largely invisible to the general public.

Explicit rationing, on the other hand, would be openly achieved by law or governmental regulation. It would therefore be visible to the entire public. Macro-rationing decisions are by definition explicit. Micro-rationing would be explicit if the law or public edict mandated which specific items of medical care would be available and for whom.

Ultimately, micro-rationing, either implicit or explicit, is required to curb the acceleration in the costs of medical care due to the increase in necessary care caused by the aging of the population and the introduction of new technology. Many people believe explicit micro-rationing to be more just than implicit rationing because it would depend upon scientific analysis, such as cost-effectiveness studies, and occur openly, and therefore, presumably would be less subject to misuse. Thus, most social scientists and medical planners prefer micro-rationing to be explicit, rather than implicitly determined by physicians.

But explicit micro-rationing has a number of procedural problems that have prevented its use. Key among these is how to determine what constitutes necessary medical care. A shortage of outcome and cost-effectiveness studies makes this determination all the more difficult. It's also unclear that people will accept any open and mandated denial of health services. However, the State of Oregon is currently considering explicit micro-rationing of medical care for some, and explicit micro-rationing is under discussion in The Netherlands.

Queuing is a less obvious but nonetheless explicit form of micro-rationing. It takes place in countries like England and Canada where global budgeting limits the availability of medical-care resources. Queuing means that patients are forced to wait for prescribed treatments that are not emergencies. Very often, the patient for one reason or another either is not treated, or else has to wait in line for an inordinate length of time. Thus expenditures for such treatments (including, most of all, new technologies) are held in check.

While affordable additional expenditure might relieve queuing, democratic governments usually are loath to increase their taxes for that purpose. Also, the affluent manage to avoid the queue by paying for private medical care out-of-pocket, either directly or most often through private insurance. Despite it's patent inequality, many planners see such turning to private care as desirable, because it both diminishes the queues, and removes those from the system most apt to complain.

While no nation has ever used explicit micro-rationing (other than by the queue), every nation uses implicit micro-rationing. Without actually making a macro-rationing decision, the United States implicitly micro-rations medical care via the marketplace, limiting entry to it and compromising on the principle of universal access in order to control its total health expenditure. Marketplace rationing's clearest result is the tiering of medical care (multiple levels of care depending upon the patient's ability to pay), but it does avoid queuing and frees doctors in private practice in the United States from the odious burden doctors have in nations with universal care: making decisions to withhold some treatments from some of their patients.

Use of copayments and deductibles, including the exclusion of drug costs from benefits, is a more subtle marketplace micro-rationing - certainly, the less affluent are far more inhibited by these tactics than the more affluent.

The other method of implicit micro-rationing is for patients' chosen physicians to make individual decisions to withhold treatment. Such decisions are obscured in this form of rationing by being made in the privacy of home or office, and within the context of individual doctor-patient relationships.

Physicians in Canada and Great Britain, both of which provide universal access and yet keep their costs to affordable levels, micro-ration implicitly. The delivery systems in these countries can be regarded as being organized to respond to professionally defined needs rather than, as in the United States, to consumer demand. Despite lesser expenditures and probably less access to many worthwhile therapies than in the United States, the Canadian and British medical-care systems enjoy broad public approval, unlike the widespread dissatisfaction in the United States. In addition, the broad indices of national health, such as longevity, infant and maternal mortality, are better in Canada and the U.K. However, that is not so when comparing the United States with other nations for quality of life and longevity according to economic status. Implicit rationing by physicians is never mentioned in nations where it is done, and its very existence has come about implicitly.

Some believe for a rationing system to be just for individuals, it has to be implemented by physicians who alone are competent to decide who needs care and is likely to benefit from it. It is contended that this form of implicit rationing achieves justice more frequently than does across-the-board application of some ideal concept.

But if physicians are to ration care justly and to the satisfaction of their patients, there are certain prerequisites. First, professional ethics based first and foremost on doctors' caring for their patients' well-being must be well established. Second, the doctor-patient relationship must be well developed. Patients must be able to relate to their physicians in a personal way, more easily accomplished with general practitioners than specialists. Family practitioners perception of their role leads them to act more like personal physicians than do specialists. In the United States only 12% of doctors describe themselves as general practitioners.

While explicit micro-rationing has never been utilized on a large scale, one such effort has been under way in the state of Oregon. Actuaries estimated the costs of 703 services. Planners then related the cost of each service to the benefit to be derived and then, after public discussion, listed each service in order of priority. Planners identified the top 587 services as basic and to be provided, leaving 122 services uncovered. The Oregon plan's objective is to shift resources away from low priority services for the 240,000 poor Oregonians currently covered by Medicaid, and instead to provide high-priority services for the estimated 120,000 poor in the state presently uncovered, who include single men, women without children and child less couples.

However, while Oregon's method to insure all 360,000 poor to a reasonable degree may seem fair, nevertheless, it has serious drawbacks.

First, the Oregon plan is too explicit about what it doesn't do. While its provisions might seem fair in the abstract, when they are applied, those denied care, along with their families and supporters, become emotional and are likely to circumvent the directives. This is known as the "rule of rescue": no matter what guidelines are set up, if a treatment is known to exist, individuals will receive it.

Second, explicit rationing plans like Oregon's often arouse irreconcilable disagreements among both lay people and experts over priority listings. (For example, a Dutch government committee of experts found that when consulting widely with the public on priorities there is need to safeguard the interests of the frail elderly and the mentally and physically handicapped).

Third, the variations in most situations are impossible to anticipate and provide just answers in advance. Consequently, fair administration of priority lists becomes difficult, if not impossible.

Finally, some look upon the Oregon principle of excluding services rather than people as wrong because 19% of the services defined as "very important" after public consultation, were excluded from the final plan.

Because Medicaid funds, the intended object of rationing, are partially derived from the federal government, federal approval was necessary to put the Oregon plan in operation. However, groups representing the disabled convinced the Bush administration that denying approval by using a patient's "quality of life" as a factor in determining the effectiveness of treatment ran counter to the American with Disabilities Act of 1990. The Oregon plan was then revised. Planners removed "quality of life" as a criterion for ranking of services. They also reduced the number ranked according to costs and benefits to 688; and raised the number of services to 568.

Some of the treatments denied would include, for example, removal of benign tumors of the skin or gastro-intestinal system, as well as treatments for low back pain, colds, obesity, infectious mononucleosis, viral hepatitis and minor head injuries. Many of the plan's included treatments are for conditions which have determined constituencies, such as AIDS, hospice care for terminally ill, Parkinson's disease, or low-birth-weight babies.

The revised plan was approved by the Clinton administration in March 1993. Oregon, already in deficit, has to find $100 million to finance the new plan.

A medical ethicist has suggested another explicit rationing method to contain costs. Daniel Callahan suggests that after a person has lived a natural lifespan, into the late 70s or early 80s, society should agree: "government should provide only the means necessary for the relief of suffering, not life-extending technology." In this context, perhaps even antibiotics might be considered such technology. This proposal is based on utilitarian criteria, including the growing burden of aged in the population, their social usefulness, and the waste implicit in the fact that 28% of annual Medicare spending is on the 6% of enrollees who die that year.

There are a number of objections specifically to using age as the criterion for explicit micro-rationing. First, people "age" at different rates: there are the "young-old" and the "old-old". Second, if we view contributions to their community as the legitimizing factor, it should be also the old-young and not only the old-old that be denied care, and this extended to the obviously futile interventions lavished on young people (especially neonates). Third, utilitarianism, the ethical basis for this criterion for rationing (and most other rationing methods, too) is not universally acceptable. Fourth, Callahan's proposal confronts the rights of mentally intact individuals to informed consent and autonomy in decision-making. Fifth, he makes passive euthanasia compulsory. Sixth, enactment would never be feasible in a democracy. And finally, if one wants to avoid the wasted Medicare expenditures at the end of life, how could one determine legally when the last year of life begins?

The U.K. and Canada use age as a criterion for rationing the more expensive medical-care procedures as, for example, dialysis, transplantation and open heart surgery. But in those countries, physicians selectively and implicitly ration using age as a criterion.

American insurers are currently trying to implement a relatively explicit rationing method, by withholding payments for specific procedures or restricting their use. However, this form of rationing has little chance of working because of the "rule of rescue": if patients or their doctors are sufficiently aggressive, they will obtain authorization for any procedure with even the most remote chance for success. The only procedures capable of firm denial are those clearly not life-saving, like artificial conception, keratotomy and cosmetic surgery. Unfortunately, eliminating such procedures has only a marginal effect on containing medical-care costs.

Alternatively, some U.S. insurance companies are using an extension of the "managed-care" concept of HMOs as a subtler form of explicit micro-rationing. This method requires approval by a specified primary physician - frequently not the patient's choice - before the company agrees to pay for a procedure. This man aged-care method makes primary physicians the balancers of a patients' interests or desire against the collective economic interest of society. Such a system under current U.S. conditions can make primary physicians and specialists adversaries in determining whether to carry out specific studies or treatments. And in an HMO the primary physician has an incentive to conserve expenditures, to enlarge the resources for his or her own remuneration.

The jury is still out on the effect of managed care on cost containment and public satisfaction. The calls for both universal medical care and cost containment are reaching crisis proportions in the United States. Certainly, if the United States is to have universal access, there must be a replacement for the current method of marketplace rationing. Explicit micro-rationing is distasteful, and probably unrealistic in a democracy. Nonetheless, the Oregon plan's explicit micro-rationing is clearly a response to the unquestionable need to equalize all citizens' access to health care. Despite the many objections to explicit rationing of medical care, does it afford a possible solution? Surely, the United States needs a demonstration project - such as Oregon's - to test the possibility.

All previous efforts by other nations to achieve universal access while containing costs have included macro-rationing by governmental budgeting of funds allocated to health care, as well as implicit micro-rationing by physicians to help hold expenditures within that budget. The British National Health Service (NHS) could provide a model for solving the U.S. medical-care crisis, but it's presently precluded because such a totally nationalized system is too radical a departure from our present free enterprise system.

However, the NHS is currently undergoing some restructuring in an attempt to overcome its too visible queuing. Results of these efforts could offer valuable insights on restructuring the American system. For example, planners are trying to increase the NHS' efficiency by forming an "internal market" for competition among providers, and by introducing some aspects of "managed care". These changes tend to make more explicit the role of physicians in offering treatment and thus, could adversely affect their ability to implicitly micro-ration. Specifically, it's important to see whether the NHS changes weaken the doctor-patient relationship, whose well-being is an important factor in the effectiveness of physicians as rationers.

Nonetheless, it's possible that the recent changes in the NHS, against the background of British macro-rationing of medical-care funding and stronger doctor-patient relationships with successful implicit micro-rationing, could be successful in the U.K., but not work to contain costs in the United States.

Many U.S. planners are endorsing adoption of a Canadian- style, tax-assisted universal health insurance plan. They suggest that if the United States would at least consolidate its myriad of third-party payers into a single payer, the savings in administrative expenses alone - upwards of 20% - would pay for the care of those presently uninsured. However, it should be noted that, over the years, Canada's containment of the acceleration in medical-care costs has not succeeded merely because of reduced administrative expenses. It has also relied upon implicit micro-rationing by physicians to stay within its macro-rationed allocation of funds.

A frequent objection to modeling a solution of the American medical-care crisis on the NHS or Canadian National Insurance system is that these are "socialized medicine". Implicit in this critique is the assumption that so-called "socialized medicine" weakens the doctor's autonomy. But for U.S. physicians or the American Medical Association to reject these models on such a basis is paradoxical, because in fact, British and Canadian physicians already practice more autonomously than U.S. physicians who submit to the conditions of managed care of HMOs, or to insurer authorizations. The majority of U.S. doctors today don't practice independently, but are employed by, for example, an HMO or a hospital. Indeed, most suggested solutions for the U.S. medical-care system include an expansion of organizations employing physicians and offering managed care, which would weaken doctors' autonomy more than modeling medical-care reform on the British or Canadian systems.

An evolutionary process of trials with various proposals will eventually determine the role of rationing in a reformed U.S. medical-care system. The paradigms from abroad, which control costs in popular systems offering universal access partly by using implicit rationing by physicians, seem to offer the most reasonable way to proceed. But, following such models may be impossible until America repairs its deteriorated doctor-patient relationship.

Unfortunately, planners, politicians and other opinion makers in the U.S. tend to ignore, or denigrate, the matter of rationing. Thus rationing will not likely enter into the discussion that will determine the shape of American medical-care reform. Yet, American success in controlling the acceleration of costs will likely be decided by whether, and how, necessary care is rationed.

Alternatively, society could decide that it would rather ignore rationing and spend an unlimited amount of its wealth on health care for everyone. However, the nation then would have to curtail and forego other forms of consumption to stay within the limits of what it can totally afford. It is most unlikely that would ever occur.

Table II-1
Rationing

1. Macro-rationing:

   A) prospective global budgets
   B) single-payer system
   C) prospective payments (DRGs)

2. Micro-rationing:

   A. explicit:

      a) by the queue
      b) Oregon plan
      c) by age

   B. implicit:

      a) by the marketplace
      b) by doctors in private practice (as abroad)
      c) managed care (in United States)

Chapter III

Health Services Abroad

All advanced industrialized countries, except the United States and South Africa, provide reasonably universal access to medical-care and yet contain their costs well below those of the United States. Countries abroad restrain medical-care costs rationing through means other than the marketplace and their populations are satisfied with their medical-care delivery systems, again in contrast to the United States Nevertheless, costs of medical care in these countries continue to escalate - although at a rate lower than in the United States - and all nations abroad are also constantly seeking ways to curb the escalation in medical-care costs.

In all nations, more affluent people can obtain as much care, as quickly as they desire by paying for it out-of-pocket, either directly or, more frequently, by purchasing supplementary insurance. Most planners view this obvious tiering of medical care as desirable, because it reduces costs to the state and mutes some of the complaints against the system.

Nationalized Comprehensive Health-care Systems

Nationalized comprehensive health-care systems are national systems funded by taxes and offering comprehensive health care to the entire population. The state sets the budget for the entire system and regulates its operation. In general, in contrast to insurance programs

- even universally mandated ones - there is no separate accounting for each service rendered the individual.

British National Health Service (NHS)

Access. Health care is available to all residents.

Financing. The government broadly regulates the delivery of health care through the NHS and funds it from general tax revenues.

Hospitals. Hospitals are owned and operated by the government and have become well regionalized under the NHS.

Physicians. The government pays for medical training; general practitioners who maintain private offices (called "surgeries" in Britain) provide ambulatory practice and are paid according to their activity. GPs receive 60% of their income from an annually-set capitation fee for each patient on their list. Forty percent of their income derives from fees for special items-of-service the government believes needs emphasis and incentive, such as vaccinations and immunizations, cervical cytology tests, contraceptive advice, inserting intrauterine devices (IUD's), maternity services, emergency treatment, and night visits. A single practitioner is limited to 3500 patients on a list, but the average list contains about 2000 patients; the ratio of GPs to population is 1 to 1758. Specialist physicians (called consultants) practice in hospitals and are on salary.

Under the NHS, patients can choose their general practitioner and practitioners can choose patients for their lists. The choosing of specialists in the U.K. traditionally (even before the NHS) had been on the recommendation of the general practitioner. Therefore, neither the public, physicians nor planners mind that patients have no direct access to specialists in the NHS. Such freedom-of-choice is somewhat illusory at any rate, since patients rarely have sufficient knowledge to make a medically beneficial choice. Further, when their need is greatest, as in an emergency or during acute illness, patients have the least ability to shop around. Even private insurance plans in the U.K., while theoretically offering a choice of specialists, thus do not increase freedom-of-choice; they do, however, make medical care more convenient and avoid the queue.

The Family Practitioners' Services account for 22.4% of the NHS budget. It also provides funds for out-patient drugs, which are responsible for 50% of this service's total expenditure. While patients contribute to their costs, dental and optical care account for 20% of the general practitioners' service budget, leaving 30% for physicians' pay. Family practice committees, after negotiation with the government ministry, govern general practice activity.

Cost containment. *Macro-rationing* - annual global budgeting for the entire NHS. The Ministry of Health sets hospital budgets and is the single payer that negotiates salaries for consultants and remuneration for general practitioners and sets the cost of drugs sold to the NHS by manufacturers.

Micro-rationing is achieved by doctors and by the practice of queuing.

Comments. Britain expended 6.1% of its GDP on health care in 1990, compared to 12.2% for the United States the same year. That percentage remained the same in the U.K. the next year, while United States expenditures rose to 13.2% of GDP.

Doctors in the U.K. earn about twice their nation's average wage or salary, compared with 2.9 times in Canada and six times in the United States British doctors' incomes have decreased by 20% in real terms since 1950. However, they have maintained their autonomy in practice, to their own professional satisfaction. Maintenance of autonomy has also allowed them to be the principal means for rationing the limited resources made available to the NHS.

There is much queuing for non-emergency services in the NHS. Patients must wait for appointments and wait in doctors' offices. They are placed on lists for elective surgery. There are two such lists - for urgent and non-urgent cases. While health authorities have ruled that urgent cases must be done within one month and the non-urgent cases within a year, in fact many patients wait well beyond these time limits. This problem motivated the Tory Government to prescribe in 1991 the radical changes described below.

This tax-based system is claimed not only to be fairer than the U.S. system, but also conducive to better national health. Payment for health costs in the United States is regressive: the poorest 10% of the U.S. population receive 1.3% of total income but pay 3.9% of health costs, while the richest 10% receive 36.8% of income and pay only 21.7% of health costs. In Britain, it is the other way around: the poorest decile receives 2.3% of income and pays only 1.7% of health costs, while the top decile receives 24.9% of income and pays 25.6% of health costs. Regressive health payments add to health costs because it has been proven that the better the income, the less there are individual health problems.

Private medical care in 1991 served about 5.5 million people or eight percent of the British population. Private Insurance in the U.K. covers only hospitals and consultants, not primary care. Many consultants (specialists) augment their in comes by practicing privately one day a week. The Official work week in the NHS is 44 hours, but most consultants work longer hours for which they are not paid. Consultants earn only slightly more than GPs, but under a "maximum-full-time-agreement" are free to work privately. This agreement obliges them to work in the NHS at least 38.5 hours per week for which they receive nine- elevenths of a full salary. Forty three percent of consultants work full-time in the NHS and another 25% work under the maximum full-time arrangement. Ten percent of consultants work entirely outside of the NHS. Specialists comprise only 20% of doctors in the U.K. (the reverse of the proportions in the United States). They do no primary care; the 80% of doctors who are general practitioners do no hospital work.

Britain's Conservative government favors privatization of care, and has made tax exempt the cost of providing private health insurance for employees who earn less than 8500 pounds per year ($13000 in 1986). Even ardent supporters of the NHS support this policy, believing it alleviates queuing, provides more convenient medical care for those who desire it, and introduces an element of competition that helps keep the NHS efficient. At the very least, it siphons off its severest critics from the NHS. About 90% of the work done in private hospitals is elective surgery; about one-fifth of these are abortions.

While the NHS has not achieved its original aim of "universalizing the best" in health care, it has succeeded in "universalizing the adequate". It has also achieved greater geographical equity in distribution of medical-care resources than any other country. NHS has achieved these goals with a remarkable containment of costs, spending the least of all countries belonging to the Organization for Economic Cooperation and Development (OECD): 5.9% of its GDP, or $842 per capita in 1989. Despite lower expenditures on medical care, the overall statistics for longevity and infant and maternal mortality, which reflect total health care, are better in the U.K. than in the United States, and the NHS is viewed with affection by the

British people, even if it limits access to some worthwhile therapeutic modalities.

Nonetheless, the British government in 1991 imposed some restructuring on the National Health Service (NHS) in an effort to eliminate queuing without any significant increase in expenditure. With advice from an American health economist, Alain Enthoven (see Chapter V, 2A), the government is attempting to increase the efficiency of the NHS by introducing competition among providers through creation of an "internal market" with the purpose of causing "the money to follow the patients". Hospitals will be allowed to "opt out" and manage their own budgets. It is anticipated that this will cause them to compete for referrals, both from health authorities and those practitioners who have their own budgets, by being more efficient and having more room for patients who, then, would not need to queue.

In addition, some general practitioners, (groups with lists of 9,000 or more) have been given their own budgeted amounts of a million or more pounds for the care of their patients. These GPs with their own budgets can make referrals to wherever they wish. After 1993 groups with lists of 7000 to 9000 patients will be permitted to hold their own budgets (fund holders). These changes put budget-holding practitioners in a similar position to American HMO doctors: they are encouraged to restrict referrals, and to look for the "best deal" when they do make referrals, both to avoid their patients having to queue and to seeking the lowest costs to their budgets. Most British practitioners opposed these changes, objecting that cost containment incentives will erode many decisions that otherwise would be made with only the best interests of patients in mind. The British physicians objected even though the money saved had to be reinvested in practice improvements, and is not retained as income, as it is in U.S. HMOs.

Many observers consider these NHS reforms, instituted by the Conservative Thatcher Government, as a step toward returning medical care to the private sector, in line with the overall Conservative policy of privatization of governmental activities. However, the issue of continued financing of the NHS has been left unresolved, and further reform of the NHS might not be necessary if tight public funding leads many of those who can afford it, to resort to privately-funded medical care.

Sweden

Access. Access is universal.

Financing. Sweden's universal health system is delivered through their county governments and is partly funded by a proportional income tax amounting to an average of 9%. Other revenue comes from an insurance fund paid into by employers for each employee.

Hospitals. Almost 100% of hospitals are state owned (through the counties) and are regionalized so that all parts of the country are efficiently served. They are financed 88% by taxation, 8% by health insurance funds and 4% by patient copayments.

Doctors. Doctors receive salaries, but the incomes of generalists (or primary physicians) are supplemented by patient fees so that doctors have incentive to see more patients. The fee to see a general practitioner was seven crowns ($1.48) in 1972, 15 crowns for a home visit and 2 crowns for a telephone call (see below under "cost containment" for 1992 fees). In 1992 incentive pay for specialists to make them more productive was under discussion. Only about five percent of doctors are solely in private practice.

Swedish patients have the freedom to choose both their general practitioner and hospital specialist. Unlike the NHS, the Swedish system allows patients to go directly to hospitals with out a referral from their general practitioner.

Cost containment. *Macro-rationing* - the central government sets an annual global budget for health care. Counties negotiate and set fee schedules for physician, hospital reimbursement and cost of drugs. *Micro-rationing* - Copayments, starting January 1992, were increased so that patients paid the equivalent of $16 to see a GP, $21 to consult a specialist in an out-patient department and $27 for treatment in an emergency room of a hospital. This scale of fees was designed also to encourage patients to use a general practitioner. The scale of these charges may surprise those used to viewing Sweden as the epitome of an advanced welfare state. The planners hoped patients would naturally prefer to see GPs rather than go directly to the hospital.

Since 1976, Sweden has had a Treatment Injury Insurance Law which establishes a money-saving, no-fault social insurance for harmful results of treatment. Patients needn't prove negligence or incompetence. A patient who can merely show some harmful effect is automatically compensated by a Medical Responsibility Board, out of insurance premiums paid by county governments.

Comments. In 1989 Sweden spent 8.8% of its GDP on health care or $1361 for each person. That compares with 11.8% and $2354, respectively, spent that year in the United States. In 1992, health care still only took 8.8% of Sweden's GDP.

Sweden is concerned about escalating costs of medical care and changes similar to those introduced into British NHS in 1991 are being tested. For example, Stockholm County has set up nine political boards with the responsibility for purchasing services, after consultation with GPs, from county public and private hospitals. Hospitals are expected to compete for con tracts. The local boards also negotiate general practice budgets, tied to population based contracts. Practitioners, in turn, negotiate contracts with local hospitals for their referrals. There are no general practice fund holders, as in Great Britain, but they are looking for ways to stimulate the productivity of their salaried doctors.

The Swedish system has evolved over the past thirty years, and is still undergoing change. Its planners have always aimed to curtail the systems steadily increasing costs by giving incentive to patients not to exploit the system, and by increasing its providers' productivity.

State-mandated Social Insurance Systems (i.e., Canada, Germany, The Netherlands, France, Japan)

These health systems are funded primarily from government mandated social insurance whose premiums are community-based, rather than experience-rated. Experience-rated premiums are set according to the expected loss in the various categories of patients. So for example, premiums are higher for smokers than non-smokers. Community-rated premiums are the same for everybody.

Enrollment in the basic social insurance plan is obligatory for workers and it covers themselves and their families. The amount of contribution varies with income. Consequently, better paid workers subsidize lower-paid workers, and the young and single subsidize the elderly and those with large families. Employee and employer share the insurance plans' contribution. For example, German automobile workers' weekly contribution is 6% of their earnings and that is matched by their employers. Employers never pays more than 50% of the premium. Everyone must purchase insurance, and the insurance funds must accept all applicants, regardless of their pre-existing conditions or occupation, or any other factor.

Social insurance plans are not free market plans. The governments exert considerable control over their operation, and play a major role in determining the premiums paid by workers and the fees paid to doctors and hospitals. There is an annual negotiation by all parties (the government, insurance plans, private insurers, hospitals, medical associations) to set the premiums, benefits and fees for the next year. This makes these systems, in essence, a single-payer one.

In many of the social insurance countries, patients directly pay something when they receive a service. It's possible, but not obligatory, to take out insurance for these copayments. Generally, no direct charge to the elderly, unemployed or chronically ill is allowed; and prolonged illness is never as expensive as it often is in the United States. Insurance funds pay for work done in hospitals on a fee-for-service basis, or by a daily rate determined at the yearly negotiation session. General practitioners usually are paid on a fee-for-service basis, but sometimes are salaried. A general characteristic of insurance programs is that each service rendered to an individual is paid for separately to the provider.

There are two varieties of social insurance systems: government administered insurance, as in Canada; and government-regulated social insurance, as in all other countries with social health insurance. The Canadian system is administratively less complex because it eliminates a management layer represented by social insurance organizations and the few purely private ones surviving in the second alternative. Both options provide universal medical care, and most have kept their costs to a level that has approximated the growth of their gross domestic product.

Government-administered Universal Health Insurance

Canada

Access. Universal coverage, including long-term care, is obtained in the Canadian system through public sector insurance administered by a provincial public agency.

Financing. The system, called Medicare, is financed by premiums from employers and employees supplemented by the federal and provincial governments from taxation. Employees typically pay about $50 a month. The federal contribution originally was 50% but has dropped since becoming tied to the growth of the Canadian GNP. In 1993 it is only 30%. Because the provinces' premium payments increases if Medicare's costs grow faster than Canada's GNP, provinces have a strong incentive to limit their expenditures. In 1987, public payments accounted for 74% of Canada's total expenditure for medical-care services; private insurance and individuals made up the balance paying for services not covered by the provincial plans. By contrast, private payers in the United States - insurance companies and individuals - provided 57% of the funds used to purchase a total of medical care in 1987 that did not cover everyone.

Hospitals. Hospitals are reimbursed for operating expenses, but not for capital costs. Each year the provincial governments' Ministries of Health forecast expected costs increases for food, labor, fuel, and other necessities. The Ministries then propose a percentage increase in reimbursements to allow the hospitals to maintain their levels of services. Individual hospital administrators then develop hospital budgets in line with their expected funding. The Ministries of Health review and approve these budgets. Administrators can negotiate justifiable increases in the hospital budget, and the ministries also can allow province-wide budget increases if their forecasts prove wrong. Since 1977, ministries have approved and allowed extra funds for new and special programs such as special cardiac, neonatal intensive care, dialysis, and chemotherapy units. Since 1979, Canada's medical education budget has funded intern and resident salaries separately.

Hospitals send no bills to patients but work from an annual operating budget. If a hospital runs a deficit, it has to be made up the following fiscal year. Hospitals therefore limit their services, resisting any extra demand and creating queues for many special services. Thus Canadians must wait for elective hospital admissions and elective surgery. The budget constraints also influence the care doctors recommend. Such implicit rationing by physicians, as in the U.K., is Canada's ultimate means of cost containment. The large proportion of doctors who are general practitioners and can attend personally to patients and establish a close and trusting relationship aids the implicit rationing process. Despite this kind of rationing and the queuing, Canadian Medicare remains very popular.

Physicians. Fees are negotiated periodically. All office visits cost the same. Thus there is no "fee schedule creep" as in the United States, where a "full and comprehensive visit" is better paid than an ordinary visit. Patients choose their own doctor, but the doctor bills the province. There is no cost sharing and physicians are generally not allowed to bill in excess of the provincial fee schedule. Diagnostic tests are centralized in hospitals and laboratories and are not allowed in doctors' offices. The fee schedule pays only for physicians' work, not for that of their employees'; the only way a practitioner can increase income is to work harder. On the other hand, there is no regulation of clinical practice, and doctors receive regular monthly payment of their fees and have no unpaid debts.

Canadian provincial governmental regulations cultivate primary care practice. Fifty percent of Canadian physicians are general practitioners; half of Canadian medical graduates select further education leading to a career in general practice (family medicine).

Cost containment. *Macro-rationing* - is accomplished by the provincial governments applying pressure on doctors' fee schedules, and on hospital costs through regulation of their physical capacities and budgets. The provinces act as the single payer when negotiating budgets with hospitals and fees with physicians. Also, if a physician exceeds a set billing amount in any one year, his or her payments are reduced in the next period to make up the difference.

This same mechanism of prospective global budgeting combined with single-source reimbursement controls the availability of new technologies. It has also permitted the government to limit the supply of hospital beds and number of hospital employees. A Patent Medicines Prices Review Board keeps the cost of drugs 30% below those in the United States. Nevertheless, in 1993 a budget deficit forced the province of Ontario to cut $195 million (20%) from its $1.1 billion Drug Benefit Plan that pays for the free drugs given to 2.4 million seniors and welfare recipients.

The administrative cost of Canada's universal health insurance program is three percent. In comparison, the administrative cost of the U.S. private insurance system is over 20%, and 16% of Americans are uninsured. In other terms, the U.S. system takes 1.23% of GDP for administration, compared to 0.1% of GDP for Canada. Estimates of administrative savings if the United States adopted the Canadian system, vary from $46.8 to $100 billion a year.

Under the Canadian system, case managers and needs - assessment specialists, mostly non-physicians, evaluate the need for long-term care and authorize payment for service. Forty to 51% needing long-term care are under 65. Federal and provincial budgets for acute and long-term care are kept separate.

Some provincial governments impose a nominal "user's fee" for hospital amenities. By 1993, planners were discussing broadening and increasing user's fees in order to reduce deficits.

Comments. Canada's universal health insurance program, established in 1970, successfully kept the cost of health care down to seven percent of their GNP for almost two decades. However, by 1991, that cost had risen to 9.2% of GNP, compared with 12.3% of GNP in the United States the same year.

Canada doesn't let price play a role in allocating medical-care resources. Instead professionals ration the care, denying treatment to some and making others wait. In contrast, the cost of dental care, uncontrolled in Canada, keeps increasing rapidly.

Some Canadian physicians and hospital administrators have attacked their medical care system, complaining it's underfunded and hence subjects the Canadian public to a shortage of physicians' care and insufficient hospital facilities and new technologies. These critics also point to waiting lists for hospital care and elective surgery, and to wealthier patients seeking services in the United States. Nevertheless, the Canadian Medical Society does not call for dismantling the system. Instead, it demands increased funding, raising it by one or two per cent of GNP.

Before the introduction of universal insurance in 1970, Canadian physicians' income increased at the rate of 4-5% per year. Since then, the increase has been about one to two percent each year. Canadian physicians' incomes increased from three and one-half times the national average in 1955 to five and a half times the average in 1971. Since 1971, this ratio has decreased. By 1980 the multiple fell to 2.9, where it has remained (in the United States, in 1992, that multiple was 6; in Germany 3.5 and in the U.K., two). But physicians are still Canada's highest-paid professionals. In Ontario, in 1991, each of its 25,000 doctors billed an average of $177,000. In 1993, however, the system's budget deficit and consequent cuts in outlay for medical care by $1 billion to $16 billion meant $4 billion to doctors and each doctor was cut $11,000.

The hospital underfunding complaint in Canada is more complex. Seventy percent of hospital operating budgets go to wages. Provincial governments, fearful of strikes, make frequent wage concessions. As a result, to stay within the budget, hospitals must limit their size and capital expenditures. Acquisition of new technology is also affected. For example, to help reduce its deficit, the province of Ontario in 1993 shrunk hospital funding by $160 million, cutting back on special programs such as dialysis and transplantation. In addition workers were forced to take 12 unpaid holidays a year.

Planners defend the constraints on technology by pointing out that in most industries, new technology reduces the unit cost of products. In medical care, however, technology is most often a source of cost increases. In the United States, since third-party payers have opted to support procedures rather than office visits to the physician, technology's expansion of the range of small procedures results in an increase of services, thus raising the incomes of health providers. In Canada, on the other hand, doctors can't benefit financially from new technology, since diagnostic tests are limited to hospitals and laboratories. Canadian planners say limiting the number of new big technological units means they are used more wisely. Such units are used more intensively than in the United States. Canadian planners believe in collecting data so that technological advances can be introduced rationally, both as to its nature and amounts. In further defense of their system, they point out that, overall, the health of Canadians is excellent and that life expectancy as well as infant and maternal mortality surpass those same measures in the United States.

By 1993, many provinces began responding to increasing costs by adopting a "community-based" model for medical care and off-loading costs onto municipal tax rolls.

Why does the United States not adopt a medical-care system based on the Canadian model? Observers say that taxes for such a system, an estimated $250 billion, are not politically feasible in the United States, even though such taxes would actually constitute a transfer from less visible spending in the private sector. Also, the American private health insurance industry, which would be eliminated, and other vested interests such as unions and suppliers, would lobby against such a change. Finally, some observers say the Canadian system is too egalitarian for the United States. The rich wouldn't want to be treated the same as the poor and would politically oppose adopting a Canadian-style system.

Government-regulated Social Insurance

Germany

Access. Eighty-eight percent of the German population are covered by not-for-profit, private insurance organizations known as sickness funds. Each of the 1147 sickness funds operates in a given area. In 1991, all workers earning less than $36,580 by law had to make contributions to a sickness fund varying from four to eight percent of their gross salary. Employers matched their contributions to the fund. If workers' incomes were above $36,580, they still could enroll in the sickness fund, but they were allowed to opt for private insurance and thus not contribute to a fund. The large number of funds is accounted for by their being organized for all varieties of groups, trades and crafts, as well as for large employers, and by locality. In addition, there are national funds for white collar, the self-employed and unemployed. The state pays the premiums for the unemployed.

The remaining 12% of the population buys private health insurance from for-profit or non-profit companies, with employers contributing toward the premium the same amount contributed for a sickness-fund member.

Financing. Sickness funds receive the income from an income-adjusted family premium, paid half by the employee and half by the employer, retirement fund or unemployment fund. Premiums for funds vary according to services provided and the actuarial-determined risk of the fund's enrollees. One fund's premium can be twice another's.

Higher earners in Germany may choose to pay higher premiums into alternate insurance plans that provide more generous bene fits. There are a few large non-profit health funds, and a larger number of private for-profit plans. Multiple plans arguably encourage competition but, in fact, only the higher earners have a relatively wide choice of insurance funds.

The government pays contributions into the basic plan for the unemployed and chronically ill. Pension plans pay contributions for the retired at the same rate as the average national payroll contribution of workers, which was 12.8% in 1991. These pension plan contributions cover only about 40% of the care of the elderly. The sickness funds pay the remainder.

Hospitals. Hospitals in Germany are 50% state owned. The rest are owned by for-profit or non-profit corporations, or by insurance plans. Hospitals receive a per diem rate for operating expenses (negotiated with the sickness fund in their locale) that is the same for all payers no matter what the diagnosis. Hospital capital expenses come from governmental funds, principally from the states who also review and approve the hospitals. Hospitals are fewer in Germany, but - as a result of 40 years of regional resource allocation planning - generally larger and better distributed than in the United States.

Doctors. Doctors are paid fee-for-service for ambulatory patients on the basis of a negotiated fee schedule. Hospital-based doctors are salaried, and sharply demarcated from the 90% who provide outpatient care and are represented in negotiations by their own association. Patients must receive a referral to see a specialist or to be hospitalized. But once having received a referral slip they're free to choose the specialist or hospital.

Cost containment. *Macro-rationing* - through prospective budgeting by a national forum, The Concerted Action in Health Care, which develops targets that frame the negotiations between insurers and providers. The federal government also participates in these deliberations. In addition, the sickness funds and insurance companies participate in a number of self-regulatory efforts through regional and national councils. However, they are regulated as a public utility, and allocate medical-care resources in a way that limits expenditures.

Under the German system much effort goes into holding down fees and ensuring that hospital budgets are not excessive. A policy of not permitting increases in insurance premiums to exceed the rise in workers' wages and salaries required the German Parliament to pass Cost-Containment Laws in the 1980s. These laws, while not significantly reducing services to patients, imposed tighter controls on physicians' fees, hospital budgets and the cost of drugs.

Since workers pay at least half the premiums, unions exert considerable pressure on doctors and hospitals to keep fees and budgets as low as possible. The budgets are set by regional yearly negotiations between organizations representing insurers and providers. This method creates, in effect a single-payer system. All providers receive the same rates and are obliged to treat all the insured.

Micro-rationing - is achieved in several ways. Some employers require copayments by patients, to reduce usage. The Cost-containment Law reforms in 1988 included expansion of copayments for drugs, durable medical equipment and dental care, which is fully covered. (At the same time, however, long-term home health care and more preventive services were added to the benefits of some sickness funds.) The patient thereafter contributed $7 a day for hospitalization, but only for a maximum of 14 days in any one calendar year; 50% of the cost of a dental prosthesis; and 15% of the cost of unlisted drugs. The insurance plans refund fully the cost of 30% prescription drugs which are listed and whose prices have been negotiated with the pharmaceutical companies.

Germany also has increased its physician education on utilization, rather than resorting to American-style peer review organization) activity. The Germans have, however, as in the United States instituted profiling of physicians' prescribing habits, and penalize those who exceed the norm.

Comments. In 1989, Germany spent 8.2% of its GDP on health or $1232 per person, as opposed to 11.8% or $2354 per person the same year in the United States. Despite the 1988 reforms holding the overall cost of health care in 1989 and 1990 to about 8% of GDP, costs to sickness funds for individuals in 1991 increased by 10%, while premium income increased only five percent. Thus, to avoid raising premiums - which in 1992 amounted to between 8% and 16.8% of income - Germany enacted a rigid 1993 budget which froze the growth of spending. This measure increased patient copayments, limited increases of doctors' salaries and fees, and hospital rates, and further limited dental and drug reimbursements. It also froze payments to drug companies and pharmacies at 1991 levels and penalized doctors for over-prescribing.

Critics of the German system object to the unwieldy number of sickness funds, and the extreme separation of hospital and ambulatory-care doctors. This separation causes hostility between the two kinds of doctors, as well as duplication of equipment and studies, and retardation of development of outpatient surgical and other specialty care. Also separate decision making by the German states, as well as by the state and central governments impedes planning, efficient deployment of resources, and cost containment.

The Netherlands

Access. In the Netherlands, 62% of the public are covered through 35 regional sickness insurance funds, in 1991 limited to those with an income of $30,000 or less. The 38% of the population with higher incomes purchase private insurance from non-profit and for-profit insurers.

Health insurance in the Netherlands is compulsory, and low income individuals receive a government subsidy to buy it. The Exceptional Medical Expenses Act of 1960 reduces insurance costs by providing anyone with unusual costs, such as those necessitated by extended or catastrophic care.

Financing. The cost of insurance and the Exceptional Expense Fund is financed by employer, and employee and self-employed contributions adjusted to incomes. The government makes contributions for the unemployed and low income people. The insurance system is administered by the sickness funds. A central fund dependent on the tax collector provides the subsidy for low income people. Premiums are based on age, sex and a variety of risk factors; exclusion of pre-existing conditions or refusal of insurance is common. Employers frequently pay 50% of the premiums for private insurance for their upper income employees.

Hospitals. Dutch hospitals charge insurers a daily rate. All are non-profit and 85% state-owned. After 40 years of central planning, they are larger, fewer and more widely dispersed than in the United States.

Physicians. General practitioners, who outnumber the specialists in the Netherlands, are paid per capita for sickness-fund patients. They treat private-insurance patients on a fee-for-service basis. The insurance plans set a target income for doctors and arrange the per capita payment arranged so as to provide 70% of it, expecting each practitioner to earn the remaining 30% from private practice.

Specialists receive fee-for-service from all patients. The patient can choose the doctor but must have a referral from a practitioner to consult a specialist. Specialists have to consult with the practitioner before referring to a second specialist.

Cost containment. *Macro-rationing* - Hospitals negotiate a global-revenue- budget annually with the sickness funds and major private insurers. The budget includes estimates of volume and kind of services, and cost factors. If the budget underestimates revenues, hospitals have to pay back the excess. If the budget over-estimates, the hospital receives extra revenue the next year. These estimates of hospital revenue are independent of costs. Thus if the hospital keeps its costs down, it can keep the profit from the estimated revenue. This approach creates incentive to operate efficiently and keep cost lean by, for example, using ambulatory rather than inpatient surgery.

A "Sickness Funds Council", made up of employer, labor union, patient, hospital, doctor, fund and government representatives, regulates the sickness funds. The government gives The Council power to monitor the funds and to negotiate, as a single payer, for doctors' fees and incomes, and drug costs.

Micro-rationing - private insurers frequently require a variety of deductibles for as much as 20% of the fees, and also give rebates for non-usage.

Comments. The Dutch system is administratively complex. The prospective budgeting system reduces innovative initiative. Health-care inflation, though always less than in the United States, has exceeded general inflation over the last two decades, although remarkably less so in the last 10 years. Health expenditures advanced from 6% of GDP in 1970 to 8.2 in 1980 and to 8.3%, or $1135 per person, in 1989. In contrast, 1989 costs in the United States were 11.8% of GDP or $2354 per person.

Dutch medical-care costs are expected to rise to 10.6% of GNP by 2005. The government has set a goal to reduce health expenditures to 8.5% by 2005. Therefore, it has partly adopted proposals of a panel of experts appointed in 1987. These proposals partly based on Enthoven's plan for "managed competition" (Chapter V - 2A), combined with a new macro-rationing one-payer mechanism to integrate the three forms of insurance into one system. The panel also recommended adding support for long-term care for the chronically ill.

Under the proposed changes in the Dutch system, the care-insurer will receive per capita budgets from a central fund, along with nominal copayments from members. Competing on the basis of nominal co-premiums, the insurers will selectively contract with providers based as much on quality as on marginal costs. The panel also proposed that monitoring care and audit activities be enhanced. However, both recent political changes in the Netherlands' government and failure to resolve discussions on necessary regulations - including agreement on a definition of "necessary care" for making explicit rationing choices - have slowed implementation of these changes.

France

Access. Since 1967 France has consolidated its many sickness insurance funds into three, regulated by the Ministry of Social Affairs and Employment. One fund is for salaried employees, and which enrolls 76% of the population. A second, for farmers and agricultural workers comprises 9% of the population, and the third fund is for the 7% who are self-employed. The remaining 8% of the population come under special welfare programs that supply health insurance administered by the Ministry of Health.

Financing. Employees contribute 6.8% of salaries to sickness funds. A majority of the French people subscribe to voluntary supplementary insurance plans to cover copayments. Local and central government provide public hospital capital costs. About one-third of such costs comes from the national health insurance organizations. While France's many proprietary hospitals are financed privately, philanthropy and church contributions, with some public funding, finance construction of voluntary hospitals.

The French insurance funds supply all hospital operating expenses, according to a negotiated prospective budget. The funds pay the hospitals a per diem flat fee, with extra fees for certain ancillary diagnostic and treatment services. Hospital costs absorb more than 50% of insurance fund expenditures.

Hospitals. Sixty-six percent are state-owned. Under The Hospital Law of 1970, each of the country's 21 administrative regions is considered a hospital service region. This has facilitated regional planning and regulation of all institutions and services, private as well as public. The system is now based on a regional hospital which is usually affiliated with a medical school and associated with a network of local hospitals.

Doctors. Patients pay general practitioners' office fees directly, and then are reimbursed for 75% of the fee by the local branch of the sickness fund. Specialists, who work full-time in hospitals, are salaried. In 1980 an estimated 30% of French physicians were salaried. To lessen the negotiating strength of the private practitioners, many local sickness funds have set up health centers with salaried doctors for ambulatory care.

Cost containment. *Macro-rationing* - since 1984, hospitals have been allocated a prospective global budgetary amount. A government committee sets drug costs a little below what they are in other countries. As a result drugs in France are the least expensive in Europe, and 60 to 70% cheaper than in the United States. However, because of public mores, the French spend more than Americans, English or Canadians on drugs and less than Germans or Japanese.

Micro-rationing - Patients must pay substantial copayments for hospitalization - 20% of per diem rates up to a 30 day maximum. Hospitals bill the sickness funds directly for the remaining 80%. However, all copayments are waived for old-age pensioners and the indigent. Ambulatory doctors' fees must conform with a negotiated official schedule.

Comments. In 1989, France spent 8.7% of its GNP, or $1274 per person, on health care. That contrasts with an U.S. expenditure of 11.8%, or $2354 per person, the same year. Despite these figures, France's health expenditures have increased at a rate far beyond its annual rise in GDP. In response, over the past decade France has frozen, and even reduced, its number of medical students, general practitioners and hospital beds. The government has also set overall budgets for public hospitals and increased cash limits on required patient copayments.

French hospital planning has not been as successful as hoped, principally because of failure to curb the growth of private clinics. French physicians stress that fee-for-service remuneration directly by the patient, in contrast to third-party remuneration, is an important factor in forging a bond between the patient.

Japan

Access. The Employees Health Insurance Law (EHI) covers all employees of industries with five or more workers. In plants with 300 or more workers, the employer established a health insurance society, of which there are about 1800. The Japanese government, through an agency in the Ministry of Health, administers health insurance for workers in plants with fewer than 300 employees.

Everyone not under EHI is covered through the government-run National Health Insurance program (NHI). Outside the social insurance umbrella, there are also public assistance medical care programs for needy or disabled persons who can pass a means test; but 99% of the Japanese had access to care through one of the two major health insurance programs: one for the occupational groups or one for general public assistance.

Financing. Employers and employees split equally insurance premiums which averages between 3 and 8% of wages. In the government-run program, the premium covers 70% of medical-care costs, with the beneficiaries picking up the remainder. Local governments also pay 70%, but receive a subsidy from the federal government for 45%. The remaining 25% is collected from each household in proportion to its resources. In 1980 this amounted to 2.6% of taxable household income.

In Japan, the private market supplies therapeutic care, which insurance programs pay on a fee-for-service basis to physicians and hospitals. The government heavily promotes preventive care services, which are most often supplied gratis at numerous health centers throughout the nation. Supported by the central and local government, these centers provide services including health screening examinations, maternal and child care, family planning, tuberculosis control, parasite control, and nutrition counseling. They are staffed by doctors on salary.

Hospitals. Hospitals are, for the most part, privately owned. Less than 6% are owned by a governmental agency. There is no hospital planning, as such, in Japan. Apparently the Japanese assume that competition will prevent any excessive hospital construction. On the other hand, a large amount of legislation reflects the government's great concern with environmental sanitation, and public and preventive health.

Doctors. Physicians in private practice provide ambulatory care. Forty-seven per cent of doctors, the vast majority GPs, practice privately. Fifty-three percent of all physicians are hospital specialists on salary. Specialists' fees are paid to the hospitals who place it into a fund from which their doctors are paid.

Cost containment. *Macro-rationing* - A committee of providers, consumers and insurance carriers, supervised by the Ministry of Health and Welfare regularly reviews hospital and physicians' fee schedules, and the cost of drugs.

Micro-rationing - by copayments being required for insurance premiums. Under EHI insurance, the employee pays a small first consultation fee and 30% of all dependents' fees for therapeutic services, with a ceiling of 30,000 yen. Under NHI rules, all beneficiaries make a 30% copayment, with a similar ceiling. (However, the 1,700 competing insurance societies often offer rebates on copayment charges to attract members.) To discourage over-utilization, NHI and EHI are raising copayment fees for services to the elderly. The government is also training more community nurses and home-care volunteers as home helpers in order to discourage use of hospital beds for the chronically disabled and elderly. And the government is also working on providing more nursing homes, day-care centers and medical facilities for the elderly.

Comment. Japan spent 6.7% of their GDP, or $1037 per person on health care in 1989. In 1992, 6.8% of GDP went for health care. Of that amount, 75% came from public sources including insurance programs, and 25% from private sources.

Despite Japan's low overall expenditure on health, the Japanese are the greatest consumers of drugs in the world. They spend $390 per capita per year, compared with $268 per capita in the United States. Drugs account for 30% of their health care expenditures, compared with 8% in the United States. This great use of drugs results from the incentive given doctors to over-prescribe by permitting them to supply and charge for drugs.

Despite their low outlay for medical care, in 1991 Japanese had the world's longest life expectancy: women's longevity was 82.5 years, men's 76.2. Japanese life expectancy increased by 30% from 1941, at which time the Japanese had the shortest longevity of all the industrialized countries.

Japanese corporations paid somewhat more than $700 per employee annually for medical care in 1992, compared with $3453 paid by American companies.

Table III-1
Health Services Abroad

1. Nationalized comprehensive health care (i.e., England, Sweden)
2. State mandated social insurance

   2A.   government administered and controlled (Canada)
   2B.   government regulated but not administered (i.e., Germany, Holland, France, Japan)

Chapter IV

Basics of Health-care Reform

Considerations That Underlie Any
Contemplated Changes

Proposals for containment of medical-care costs entail the possibilities of more governmental regulation as well as more competition in the medical-care delivery system. These two possibilities represent two opposing ideologic poles: the first, a totally nationalized system, like the British National Health System; the second, an unregulated, free-enterprise health system (which does not exist in any advanced industrialized nation). The current American system is a compromise between these two poles, where most changes contemplated for the foreseeable future would leave it. Theoretically, placing the support of American medical care on a more purely market basis, attempting to contain costs through competition among providers, would be least disturbing. Nevertheless, the opposite approach - greater socialization of the health system in an attempt to contain costs through increased government ownership and regulation - isn't necessarily incompatible with American economic ideology. Any government, even one principally based on a free-market system, provides some services in a monopolistic or collectivist manner. For example, the U.S. government provides a defense organization, mail service, energy, water supply and irrigation projects, road and bridge construction and maintenance, as well as preventive public health services. If experience with marketplace reforms (see Chapter V, 2-A), leads us to consider therapeutic medical care as a national asset needing delivery through a fully regulated and controlled system, we should not see such delivery as a threat to the free-enterprise basis of our economy. In fact, a nationalized health system with its method of rationing might be the best way to contain the acceleration of medical costs threatening our entire economy, and in that case such a socialistic measure might be the best means to preserve our otherwise free-enterprise system.

Changes Toward More Free-Enterprise (more competition)

Most of the currently proposed programs (including those of both Republicans and Democrats) to resolve the U.S. medical-care crisis promote increased free-enterprise.

During the 1992 presidential campaign, the Democratic Party and then-Governor Clinton adopted a more centrist position than the Republican. They proposed achieving universal access both by means of private enterprise - requiring that employers provide employees with health insurance via private insurance companies - and by creating a public agency to insure those not otherwise covered. Employers could also choose to contribute a payroll tax to the public agency rather than providing private insurance for their employees. This is the essence of the so-called "play-or-pay" program.

The Democratic Party-Clinton proposals for cost-containment also included many concepts for enhancing competition in medical care delivery. Late in the campaign, Clinton proposed a cap on spending through prospective global budgeting. Nevertheless, the conservative wing of the Democratic Party, including as many as 60 national legislators in August, 1992 endorsed the Enthoven program, also called the Jackson Hole initiative, (see Chapter V, 2-A). This initiative calls for mandated employer-provided health insurance and managed competition. This latter concept was first proposed by Paul Ellwood in 1970 to the Nixon administration, and later developed by Alain Enthoven.

The Republican Party advocated on the one hand, changing tax incentives to induce more companies and individuals to use private health insurance, and on the other, giving low-income people vouchers to purchase it. Republicans did not mention a public vehicle for making health insurance available, nor did they detail their suggestions for cost-containment early in the 1992 campaign. However, in mid

1992, President Bush endorsed "managed competition" and "managed care" (the Enthoven program, also called the Jackson Hole initiative) as the means to control costs, along with tort and administrative reforms.

Proponents of using marketplace techniques such as co-pay or deductible features in prepaid insurance or government entitlement programs say they would contain costs by reducing consumer demand without direct government interference. The lowered consumer demand would make providers lower their fees. Since excessive hospital beds would not be reimbursable, the hospitals would lower their costs by reducing their unused capacity.

The concept of "managed care" (see Chapter I) also aims to control costs and yet maintain a marketplace orientation. In HMOs, managed care keeps costs down by giving doctors the financial incentive of protecting or enhancing their own incomes by limiting expenditures in the care of their patients. As practiced by insurers, proponents say managed care leads the insurance companies to dictate what is appropriate - or more often not to reimburse for what they deem to be inappropriate - in patient care.

Critics say that HMOs managed care makes physicians substitute their profits for their professional autonomy and ethics in the care of patients. Also, critics say that managed care in any form gives insurers and provider plans incentive to screen out people who need expensive care. Such screening diminishes the benefit of price competition, since it may lower costs, but only by leaving the care of more costly patients to others. Insurers' or managed-care organizations seeking to cover only "good risks" is called "cherry-picking".

"Managed competition" is a recently proposed marketplace approach to cost-containment. Under managed competition, large employers or a government agency, which are knowledgeable and represent enough potential patients to be a potent force, are given financial incentive (see Chapter I) to negotiate with providers of medical care as to costs and number and quality of services with medical care providers. These choices are not left to uninformed, or unmotivated, or weak individuals or companies. Proponents say that the resulting competition among plans offering services to patients will lower costs, or at least contain them. This is the concept of Alain Enthoven, an influential planner, some of whose suggestions have been used recently to reform the British National Health Service, and in 1992 were under consideration by the Dutch.

The recent victories internationally of free-enterprise economies over governmental centrally-planned ones confers added credence to marketplace-oriented medical-care reforms. However, one objection to enhancing the marketplace approach is that its attack on the problem of universal access is necessarily more tentative - in the sense of delayed and uncertainty of results - than the direct effect of more nationalization. Marketplace reform has never been utilized anywhere, so they have no supporting track record. The British reforms of its National Health Service along these lines are too recent for a meaningful evaluation.

Another objection to strengthening the marketplace system in medical care is that it encourages providers to provide services not according to need but according to financial return. This tendency limits the access to care by the larger and poorer portion of society. Also, competition among HMOs for subscribers often means competitive advertising and battles over turf or market share, not price-cutting. Where there are captive populations, as with Medicaid patients, HMOs have reduced costs, but often by exclusions, dis-enrollments, and reducing the quality of care.

An oft repeated objection to marketplace reforms is that favoring more competition in medical-care delivery assumes that consumers can evaluate their medical needs and thus control the demand side of the market. However this is not so. Not only does the general public lack the technical information to evaluate their own health requirements, but also most people can't be emotionally reasonable in the matter of their own medical care. Even physicians are said to be "their own worst doctor", and patients who are sick, or facing an emergency, do not have the inclination or time to shop around for care. Also distorting the medical-care market are third-parties between most consumers and providers which eliminates the immediate cost as a consumer constraint. Proponents of marketplace reforms answer that there are enough sophisticated consumers to set a proper pattern for the general public. They also offer the concept of "managed competition" as an answer to objections.

Prospective payments, such as managed care (HMOs and IPAs) for doctors and DRGs for hospitals, were primarily introduced to control costs by changing incentives for providers. However, some believe they also work to increase competition in medical-care delivery. HMOs and hospitals do compete among themselves in recruiting subscribers and patients.

On the other hand, critics of managed-care plans say they restrict patients' freedom to choose in picking their physicians, hospitals and services. Since "freedom-of-choice" is a key principle of free-market proponents as well as liberals devoted to individual rights, entrepreneurs, including physicians, and social planners (who tend to be more liberal collectivists) both fault these plans for not providing freedom-of-choice.

Managed-care plans, also, tend to interfere with patients' "continuity-of-care". Continuity-of-care means that a patient remains under one doctor's care. Continuity-of-care is not only more satisfying to patients but it is also less costly. Research shows that patients seen by various practitioners had more studies done on them, more emergency admissions to hospitals, and longer stays in hospitals. They are also less satisfied with their care than patients who stay with one doctor.

Finally, a most cogent criticism of increasing competition to contain costs in medical-care delivery - which also applies to managed care, and of administrative and tort reforms - is that while such measures can reduce costs by eliminating much unnecessary care, they cannot reduce the rate of acceleration due to the increase in "necessary care" created by aging of the population and new technology. That critique holds true so long as the basic delivery system lacks any rationing method other than the marketplace, and that marketplace method is blunted by efforts to achieve universal access. What is required, then, is some other form of micro-rationing.

Changes in a Collectivist Direction (More Regulation; or Toward a National Health Program)

Most importantly, a nationalized health program would assure universal availability. Second, placing medical care more under the government aegis makes cost containment more certain. This is because nationalization of the health delivery system, even only, as in Canada, of the insurance system, assures that there be a "single-payer system" across the board. Such a system strengthens the payer's position in negotiating budgets and fees with hospitals and doctors. In a nationalized system, physicians wouldn't have free-enterprise incentives to maximize their in comes, since they would be salaried or have their fees controlled. Physicians would have no financial reason for excessive testing, unnecessary treatments or operations, or for prolonging hospitalizations.

A national health program would not, however, compromise physicians' autonomy. In Great Britain and Canada, physicians manage their own offices and treat patients without any rules or guidelines beyond those dictated by their training, experience and professional ethics. Constraints on who gets treatment, and how much, is implied, but not dictated. Doctors micro-ration the treatments they offer their patients, limited by their availability under the national global budget set for medical care (see Chapter II).

Government control over a national health program means that prospective budgets will guarantee containment of hospital costs. It also helps achieve rational disposition of facilities, since hospitals wouldn't have the financial incentive to compete with each other. There would be no impetus to sponsor expensive public relations activities, including advertising, which increases public demand for medical care. Proponents also believe nationalized health systems respond to professionally-defined needs rather than consumer demand.

A great objection to nationalizing medical care is that physicians would become less productive, making therapeutic care less available. Critics cite as proof the long lines for elective operations, innovative tests, and even for some appointments in countries with nationalized forms of medical-care systems. Furthermore, since governments are invariably under economic constraints, they tend to under-fund a health system which has no other recourse for financial support. This underfunding causes decreased availability of new technology. Similarly, governmental efforts to pare the work force add to the inefficiency already existing due to lack of incentive.

Proponents of national health programs respond that the excessive cost of physicians' services in the United States far exceeds any financial loss that would ensue from any loss of physician productivity under a nationalized system that would restrict physician incomes. Moreover, it is not clear how detrimental to national health would be the decreased availability of therapeutic care to the affluent. Reducing the open-ended opportunity of the affluent to exploit medical care might be desirable since medical services should respond to need, rather than to demand. Anyway, studies have shown that socio-economic status is a far more powerful determinate of health than simply more and better access to medical care.

While no one questions the shortage of new technologies in Britain, their overuse in the United States is equally clear. For example, while an evaluation of renal dialysis in the U.K. showed that fewer end-stage renal failure patients were being treated than was humane. But the unlimited availability of treatment of such patients in the United States has revealed that it is overdone, being used in the most hopeless situations.

Secondly, while queuing is deplored, some planners regard it as a form of consumer restraint, ameliorating the tendency to over-utilize a free system. They point out that even an insurance-based system is "zero-priced" like a nationalized one, since there is no cost at the time of entry. In an NHS-type system, however, the increased demand generated by the zero-priced system is offset by the rationing of the available supply when physicians make decisions for individual patients (implicit micro-rationing). In contrast, American providers are reimbursed open-endedly, perpetuating the tendency for over-supply for the insured, without increasing care for those uninsured.

Even in systems less nationalized than England's NHS, the government can require all providers to be subject to the same rate-setting system, regardless of whether there is one or multiple payers (as in Germany). Such a system depends on the government controlling prices paid to doctors, hospitals and other providers.

No one is currently proposing complete nationalization of the U.S. medical-care system, like the British system. But, there are several serious proposals, including some introduced into Congress by Democrats, which advocate nationalizing health insurance, as in Canada.

Methods for Reforming U.S. Health-care System

For universal access.

There are four methods for achieving or approaching universal access: (1) with a single national health insurance plan supported by taxation, as in Canada, or by expanding the present United States. Medicare program to cover everyone, regardless of age; (2) requiring by law that all employers provide private health insurance for their employees, and providing insurance for the unemployed and self-employed through government programs; (3) providing incentive, through tax credits and tax deductions, for all individuals to buy private health insurance with the government subsidizing premiums for low-income people; (4) enacting a federally-funded national health program, as in Great Britain. (This last possibility, fully nationalizing the delivery of medical care, has neither been deemed politically feasible nor proposed by anyone.) When insurance is utilized to broaden access to medical care, its premiums can be experience-rated (or risk-rated or actuarial rated). Such a rating of premiums gives policyholders optimal value for their money and is fairer to those who are at less risk. Experience-rated health insurance is the predominant type in the United States. Alternatively, insurance premiums can be community-based (or universally rated) which means they are set by the costs of insuring masses of people, without regard to individual risk such as age, sex, occupation or previous health status. Community-based insurance premiums broaden access by making insurance accessible to higher risk groups at the expense of those at low risk. However, since those at lower risk are far more numerous than those at high risk, the increase in rates is spread widely, and therefore not too onerous.

While five percent of the American population incurs half of all medical-care expenses, and only 10% of the population incurs 70% of all expenses, most of the reform programs proposed by Democrats or Republicans (see Chapter V), nevertheless, insist on community-rated insurance. It is advocated in order to broaden access to care, and prevent loss of insurance with change of jobs because of a record of prior illness.

Of course, tax-supported national medical-care systems which provide universal access spread the costs throughout the population, with those paying more taxes supporting those paying less, or none. The indirectness of the charges, especially when the health system is supported by the general taxing system - without there being a directly labeled "health tax" - generally prevents objections to community-rated insurance premiums. Expansion of access to insurance (even if only by requiring community-rating of premiums to be) increases spending on medical care, therefore most such programs incorporate measures to control, or even reduce expenditures.

For cost containment

There are two basic approaches and several secondary methods to contain costs in the delivery of medical care. All the proposed programs for reforming the U.S. medical-care system (Chapter V) utilize one of the two basic approaches, and some of the secondary methods.

Basic methods. *Macro-rationing* is one means of cost containment. Price and wage controls are forms of macro-rationing. A single-payer system is a way of subtly imposing wage and price controls. In a single-payer system, providers are paid by a single entity, or by multiple payers, such as insurers, acting in unison. Negotiations (as in Canada and Western Europe) or unilateral fiat (as by Medicare in the United States, or U.K.'s NHS) determine reimbursements to providers. The single-payer system is also administratively less complex.

A single-payer system is usually combined with another macro-rationing stratagem, global budgeting. Global budgeting means prospectively allocating an amount of funds to medical care, often referred to as "expenditure caps". Global budgeting does put limits upon payments to providers, even when they are subject to negotiations. Prospective global budgeting is viewed by its proponents as a means of curtailing only unnecessary treatment, nevertheless, where it is used, it always requires micro-rationing of necessary care to keep expenditures within budget.

To be fully effective, global budgeting requires a nationwide single-payer system. In the United States, global budgeting could be imposed only on government-paid programs without controversial, possibly unconstitutional, legislation. Government programs account for only 43% of total health expenditures (29% on Medicare and Medicaid plus 14% on other health-programs). The private sector accounting for 57% of expenditures, urgently needs cost- containment too. The single-payer system creates as much as 20% savings by reducing administrative complexity. While administrative savings reduce overall costs substantially and global budgeting sets a target for spending, other factors causing escalation in medical-care costs continue to operate. Therefore, abroad, permanent restraint of undue escalation of medical-care costs has required that micro-rationing accompany the use of the single-payer and prospective global budgeting methods.

It is important to note that any prospective payment plan is a form of macro-rationing. Pre-payment to health plans, by capitation to an HMO or prospective payments to hospitals according to the admitting diagnosis (DRGs), gives incentive to providers to reduce, or minimize the supply of care. Opponents of global budgets and a single-payer system with price and wage controls claim that they inhibit innovations or prevent their prompt and sufficiently wide introduction into medical practice. Opponents also say limiting doctor incomes could reduce their productivity.

Since prospective global budgeting and negotiated payment schedules require micro-rationing, antagonists to these two measures attack with a mere pejorative reference to rationing. Finally, those who favor minimal governmental intervention in economic matters - a position recently buttressed by the demise of the socialist economies - oppose these macro-rationing procedures as unnecessary governmental intervention.

Increased competition - Every current proposal for battling the excessive cost escalation in the U.S. medical-care system includes the use of increased competition among providers. Since this method has never been tried anywhere in the world, its efficacy for containing costs is unproven - all the more so if accompanied by measures to attain universal access. However, some moves toward increased competition were introduced into the British NHS in April, 1991. Their effects should be measurable in 5 or 6 years.

Proponents of increasing competition in the medical-care market believe that limiting the tax free amount of premiums will give employers and patients incentive to choose the least costly insurance. They also expect that the competition to enroll these patients will both keep provider charges under control and improve their quality. Capping the amount of premiums that are tax-deductible would cause employers and patients to choose the less costly managed-care plans (HMOs, PPOs) over the more expensive fee-for-service plans. Only the least costly plans (such as HMOs) would be tax deductible. If consumers and employers seek out the least costly care, government will not have to regulate doctors' or hospital fees; competition will accomplish control by forcing providers to join or cooperate with organizations like HMOs that will gain customers by their efficiency and lower costs.

Opponents of the increased competition approach doubt that individuals are sufficiently knowledgeable to make rational medical-care choices. They fear that adequate care would be sacrificed to cost, and that entrepreneurs would find ways to keep total expenditures in the health industry escalating. In other words, the free-enterprise method of increasing competition to control costs and improve quality will not work in medical care because the product has a singular characteristic: it is perceived with difficulty by the individual consumer.

The leading proponent of increasing competition in the delivery of medical care, Alain Enthoven (see Chapter V, 2A) has offered the concept of "managed competition" to answer the objection that medical care is a "singular product". He recommends that large employers or agencies, which he calls "sponsors", who can be knowledgeable as well as powerful because of representing large numbers of patients be given incentives or be required to negotiate costs and quality of services with medical care providers. This approach would take choice away from uninformed, unmotivated, or weak individuals or companies. The notion of managed-care plays a complementary and essential role in the managed-competition proposal. Both concepts aim to replace the traditional fee-for-service, autonomous practice of physicians.

Another frequent suggestion for improving the function of the medical-care market, and curtailing the amount of care consumed, is to spend more on studies on the efficacy, or outcomes, of various treatments and disseminating the results of these studies. This suggestion aims to reduce the number of questionable treatments and eliminate those which are futile. It would include analyses of individual doctor practices, reviewing their utilization of the various methods of diagnoses and treatment. Presumably, making this information widely available would improve consumers performance in the marketplace.

Other (or Collateral) Methods. *Micro-rationing* includes several "collateral" methods to reduce usage by the insured care. One such method is to require that individuals pay a part of their insurance premium up front, thereby giving them incentive to seek out the least expensive plan. Of course, consumers may not always seek out an adequate plan - especially if they perceive themselves as young and healthy.

Another method is to require copayment at the time service is rendered, or require out-of-pocket payments for whole items, such as drugs. Alternatively, patients might have to pay limited amounts before becoming eligible for benefits - i.e., deductibles - before becoming eligible for benefits.

Requiring individuals to pay part of premiums, or deductibles, could result in tiering of care. In other words, the affluent might not cut down on medical care, but the less affluent would be induced to give up too much care. Despite studies which have shown that these methods effectively reduce usage, it is not at all clear that they eliminate only unnecessary or frivolous usage. Co-payments and deductibles has been widespread in the United States for years. While they undoubtedly reduce demand for medical care, they have not by themselves succeeded in control ling cost escalation.

Another prominent cost-control technique is "managed care" (see Chapter I), including physician profiling. Physician profiling is a euphemism for a form of micro-rationing. Whether used by insurance companies to oversee doctors' practices or effected by HMOs and PPOs, physician profiling lowers costs by giving providers a financial incentive to supply as little treatment as possible. The hope is that the only care eliminated would be needless or futile. (see Chapter I).

Operational reforms - Final collateral methods for cost containment. One such reform already mentioned which results from the single-payer system: simplification of administrative procedures, currently estimated to cost $40 to $90 billion annually, includes reduction of paper-work. Even with multiple payers, it is conceivable that forms could be unified and operational procedures coordinated so as to curtail expenses, both for insurers and providers. Administrative expenses of both the Canadian medical-care system, and Medicare in the United States are as much as 20% lower than those of the entire U.S. health-care system, proving that cost containment through administrative reform is a feasible objective in the United States.

A second proposal for modifying the operation of the health system is tort law reform. Such reform aims to decrease the expense created by litigation and the consequent practice of "defensive medicine", which costs more than $15 billion per year. In addition, doctors' and hospitals' malpractice premiums cost $14 billion annually.

Doctors and their representatives want national tort reform to follow the 1975 California Medical Injury Compensation Recovery Act. California's reforms consist of caps on non-economic damage, limits on lawyers' contingency fees, periodic payment of damages over $100,000, proportionate rather than joint and several liability, two year statute of limitations for filing most malpractice claims, and pretrial screening of claims by a medical expert. Proponents of managed competition favor tort reform through "enterprise liability". Enterprise liability would shift responsibility for negligence from individual doctors to the health plans that oversee medical-care delivery and employ doctors. Enterprise liability would not be of benefit to physicians in private practice. Enterprise liability wouldn't save the health system money, but it would cut tort system administrative cost, remove HMO doctors' fear of malpractice claims and reduce their defensive medical practice. It would give managed-care enterprises more incentive for quality control in their delivery of care.

Many analysts also propose eliminating incentives for specialization (see Chapter II) and encouraging more primary care since general practitioners provide less expensive care.

It has been stated that the savings from these operational reforms alone could immediately pay for expansion of medical care to all American citizens, without requiring additional revenues.

Of course, many of the proposed programs for resolving the medical-care crisis also include continuation and often expansion of the many previous incremental efforts to increase access and control costs (see Chapter I). There is no question that most, if not all, of these methods will lower costs of medical care. However, their proponents don't recognize that programs depending on concepts such as managed care, increasing competition among providers, administrative savings, or tort reform will not entirely eliminate the escalation in medical-care costs. They will only lower the set-point, from which escalation will continue. That's because these reforms concentrate on reducing or eliminating unnecessary care, but don't limit the acceleration in costs of "necessary care" created by aging of our population and innovations in medical care.

Table IV-1
Methods for Reforming U.S. Health-care System

A. To Achieve Universal Access

    (a) Tax incentive for private health insurance with vouchers for the poor

    (b) Mandated employer health insurance plus public agency for health insurance

    (c) National health insurance

    (d) Federally funded national health system

B. For Cost Containment

    (a) Macro-rationing

        1) single-payer system
        2) global budgeting
        3) prospective payments for services (DRGs, HMOs)

    (b) Increased competition

        1) managed competition: tax incentive to opt for least expensive provider plan by knowledgeable sponsors
        2) outcome and cost-effectiveness studies: to aid consumer choice in marketplace

    (c) Collateral methods (micro-rationing)

        1) copayments and deductibles
        2) managed care

    (d) Collateral methods (operational reforms)

        1) administrative simplification
        2) tort reform
        3) remove incentives for physician specialization

Table IV-2
Managed Competition
(financial incentives via tax system)

1. large employers: only 80% of premiums deductible makes them choose least expensive of competing "qualified" plans
2. small employers: grouped into public sponsors to get community rates; sponsors large enough to create competition among provider plans
3. Individuals: paying non-deductible 20% of premiums would choose least expensive among competing plans
4. Providers(doctors and hospitals): to compete, would be forced to join HMOs or PPOs (since they provide the least expensive care & have most patients)

Table IV-3
Managed Care

1. group HMO: prospective payments to doctors gives them incentive to conserve on care
2. staff model HMO or PPO: administrators monitor doctors on amount of care given
3. insurers: insist on prior review of care by doctors (before reimbursing patient)

Chapter V

Programs for Reform of U.S. Health-care Delivery System

Programs for reforming the U.S. medical-care system fall into four categories according to the degree of change proposed from the current system. There's also a fifth category, a program of full nationalization as in Great Britain, but no one is proposing that for the United States.

The smallest departure from our present system contemplates extending insurance coverage to those now without through tax credits. Such proposals would extend tax credits - premium costs subtracted from taxes, dollar for dollar - to those not in poverty. The poor would receive vouchers to pay their premiums. New rules for private insurance practices would stabilize insurance coverage for those already insured. These new rules would prevent "locking-in" or denying coverage to employees due to previous illnesses or pre-existing conditions. Also, small businesses would be urged to pool together and become eligible for community-rated premiums for their employees. These proposals essentially constituted the program of the Republican Party going into the 1992 presidential election. However, by mid-summer of 1992, President Bush had joined with many Democrats to support, in addition, the "managed-competition" concept.

A second category would approach universal coverage by combining employer-based insurance with health insurance supplied by a new public agency or by expansion of Medicare. Included in this group is the proposal for managed competition and managed care assembled over the past 20 years by Alain Enthoven and now called the Jackson Hole Group initiative. In September 1992, the 60 member Conservative Democratic Forum of the House of Representatives supported a bill identical to the Enthoven pro gram, plus tort reform. Also in this second category are the play-or-pay programs supported by most Democratic Party leaders. Late in his campaign for the Presidency, Governor Clinton added global budgeting to his play-or-pay package and mentioned his support for managed competition.

Listed with the play-or-pay programs constituting category two are examples of state programs already in place that mandate employer-provided insurance and/or set up public sponsors to insure those not covered by employers. These state legislations, often, were put in place in anticipation of a national initiative in this direction.

The third and fourth categories include proposals to replace the current private insurance system with a government-operated national insurance program. Programs in the third category are modeled on the Canadian system; those in the fourth category would expand the present U.S. Medicare system into the vehicle for universal national health insurance. These two categories propose the most radical departures from the current system, both for attaining universal coverage and containing costs.

Market Reform Programs (Tax Credit to Purchase Private Insurance)

Market reform programs are based on the belief that powerful incentives provided by current tax legislation are the cause of the problems of the present U.S. health system.

Most families receive medical insurance as an employee fringe benefit, not included in their taxable income. The self-employed receive limited tax relief only if they incur unusually heavy medical expenses. Consequently, for most Americans, a company plan is the only way to receive a tax break. But excluding company medical-care premiums from taxes leads to non-insurance and inflation of health costs for several reasons.

First, this exclusion is very beneficial to the higher earning employees, who get the more expensive plans. On the other hand lower paid workers with families, since they pay little or no tax, receive no tax benefit at all. But the worker with no company plan, who pays for insurance with after-tax dollars, fares worst of all. Thus the current system gives higher-paid people big tax subsidies, and no tax benefits to those at the bottom of the earning ladder. Therefore three fourths of the uninsured - those without private insurance but ineligible for Medicaid - are lower paid workers. Second, since employees don't pay for their insurance, they have no incentive to be economical when seeking services. Third, far from having any incentive to hold down costs, providers have an incentive to inflate their services and charges.

The above problems with the current system of taxing medical insurance demonstrates the benefits that would accrue from giving tax credits to purchase private insurance.

There are, in addition, several other reasons to grant tax credits for buying private insurance. Such a change augments rather than replaces the current system. it expands coverage to the uninsured and eliminates exclusions for pre-existing conditions. It would stimulate people to look for the best plans and spur insurance companies to compete to provide the most attractive coverage. This approach also avoids direct federal regulation of the fees charged private patients by doctors and hospitals.

On the other hand, while the tax credit programs would supply sufficient health insurance to more than half of those currently uninsured, the vouchers and tax credits offered to the poor, and to those with incomes up to 200% of the poverty level, would not be enough to buy adequate insurance coverage. Nor do these programs deal with the costs of long-term care. Finally, the tax credit programs suffer from the same two problems that dog many other solutions. Despite their proponents endorsement of managed care, and tort and administrative reforms, the tax credit programs don't attack the escalation in medical-care costs due to the increase in necessary care resulting from aging and new technology. And it is unclear that those given funds to buy health insurance have enough know-how to shop around. Without assistance, say critics of these programs, the average American cannot use these funds wisely.

Nevertheless, President Bush, in his 1992 campaign for re-election adopted the tax-credit approach as his answer to the medical-care crisis. Most small business representatives also support these tax-credit proposals rather than play-or-pay ones.

1-A.   Tax Reform Strategy to Deal with the Uninsured
        (program proposed by the Heritage Foundation)

To increase access. The Heritage Foundation proposes to replace the present tax exclusion strategy with refundable tax credits for health expenses. That means that if a family's tax credit exceed ed their income taxes due, the family would receive a cash refund. Employee health packages would become taxable. If a company scaled down or discontinued its health plan, it would have to add the cash value of the plan to its employees' pay checks. Employees would receive a tax credit for family medical-care costs, including insurance premiums and out-of-pocket costs. The size of tax credit, which would be refundable, would depend on the family's total health expenditure compared with its income. Finally, the tax credit system would be designed so as to ensure that the net costs for medical care would not exceed 10% of family income. One survey has shown that, presently families earning less than $12,000 pay 10.1% out-of-pocket for health expenses and this falls to 2.5% for those earning more than $20,000.

A "Health Care Social Contract" would be established. This contract would oblige all individuals and families to enroll in a health plan whose minimal provisions would include a federally-prescribed basic package, including catastrophic insurance. Payment for this plan, including deductibles, would be limited to 10% of gross income. The federal government would underwrite further expenses with either refundable tax credits or by granting access to Medicare or Medicaid.

Financing. The uninsured would be covered at no net increase in the federal deficit by replacing current tax exclusions for company-based health plans with a flat 20% income tax credit for insurance costs up to $250 per month for families and $100 for individuals. This change would collect an additional $89.4 billion in net income and payroll taxes over 5 years. It could be expanded by additional credits of $18 billion per year to cover all uninsured and still remain budget neutral.

In an attempt to reduce Medicaid and welfare costs, Heritage Foundation's proposal would give low-income people refundable tax-credits, eliminating the current disincentives for welfare recipients who receive Medicaid, to take a job with few or no medical benefits.

It would also offset government-aid costs by basing the tax-credit on medical expenses as a proportion of income, not on the family's tax rate.

Cost containment. The tax credit proposal for buying private insurance would increase competition. It would curb rising health costs because the credit system would impel patients to seek the best value for their money and avoid over-utilization. They would receive any savings they realized in cash. The incentive would be greatest for those eligible for only a small credit, generally the more healthy and affluent ones; and weakest for those eligible for a large tax credit. Employees would not be locked into the employer's plan, but could shop around, thus intensifying competition among the insurers and providers. Individuals would undoubtedly form purchaser groups, which would negotiate the most advantageous and economical plan for the group.

Administrative overhead would be reduced in a tax-credit program.

Comment. The Heritage Foundation tax credit proposal for buying health insurance would solve the problem of the currently uninsured, whether employed or not. Everyone would have at least a basic package of medical care, paid for by themselves or by the federal government.

This plan would also end both the problem of employees' "locked-in" to current jobs because of their health, and employers' hesitancy to hire because of health or age.

The average American would be protected in choosing a health plan, since all plans would be required to offer at least a basic package of services.

Finally, cross-subsidizing through the tax-code rather than through premium setting could solve the problem of younger and healthier people opting out and thus making any plan more expensive for the higher-risk.

The Heritage Foundation is politically feasible because it is less radical than replacing the entire U.S. system, as with a Canadian-style one. Also, it could be introduced gradually, covering one segment of the uninsured at a time.

1-B. President Bush's Program

In February 1992, then-President Bush endorsed a medical care reform plan which was essentially "The Equity and Access Improvement Act of 1991 (S 1936)" introduced by Senator Chafee (R, RI) to the 102nd Congress in November 1991.

To increase access. Private insurance would continue to provide medical-care coverage for most Americans.

The Bush/Chafee program, however, would give vouchers to an estimated 24.8 million low-income people not served by Medicaid. The vouchers would cover enrollment in a basic benefits plan (not including catastrophic or long-term care coverage) approved by the states. A family of three or more earning below poverty level ($13,400 for a family of four in 1992) would receive a voucher worth $3750 to purchase medical insurance.

In addition, 13.2 million people earning slightly above the poverty level would be eligible for tax credits.

An additional 56.8 million people with incomes up to $80,000 would receive a tax deductions for health insurance premiums paid out-of-pocket. The maximum tax deduction would be $3750 ($1,050 value) for a family with children, $2500 for a couple and $1250 for a single person. People with incomes above $50,000, single parents with incomes over $65,000 and couples with incomes over $80,000 would not be entitled to deductions. People receiving employer-subsidized health insurance would receive smaller tax breaks, or none at all.

Self-employed tax-payers, who in 1992 could only deduct 25% of the cost of their health insurance, would be allowed to deduct the entire amount, regardless of income.

States would be required to pass laws that would forbid insurance companies to deny coverage to individuals be cause of pre-existing conditions, or to small businesses or industries now black-listed. Charging different rates for businesses in the same industry would also be illegal.

This plan would encourage small businesses to band together to buy medical insurance for their employees at community rates, thus lowering their premiums.

Financing. The cost-containment provisions of the Bush/Chafee plan would pay an estimated one-fifth of the plan's tax breaks, which would cost approximately $35 billion annually, and the Republicans and the plan's proponents did not say how the remaining four-fifths would be met.

Cost containment. *Macro-rationing* - The Bush/Chafee plan would cap Medicaid payments for acute care. It would also cut some Medicare payments, such as to teaching hospitals, and expand limits on physician self-referral.

Micro-rationing - This program would give incentive to all Americans, but especially the poor, to join managed-care plans like HMOs, because they would be able to keep the savings from joining cheaper plans. Under this program, employer and employee contributions would establish medical-care accounts for buying health insurance or individually purchased services. Since individuals could keep unspent after-tax amounts, they would have an incentive to avoid unnecessary usage.

Increased competition - To help consumers make better choices states have to publish hospital, doctor and laboratory charge, and rate their comparative quality and outcome data.

Tort reform - The plan would change medical malpractice laws by giving incentives for arbitration, limiting pain and suffering payments to $250,000.

As an addendum to the Bush/Chafee plan, Senator Bond, at President Bush's request, introduced in June 1992 a bill to save administrative expenses. The Medical and Health Insurance Information Act of 1992, would require electronic submission of all insurance claims after January 1, 1994 and computerization of hospital medical records by 1996. It would establish a framework for administrative reform, requiring continuing consultation with private groups to develop its details. If the private sector did not complete its rules for electronic claims transmission and computerizing record-keeping, the Department or Health and Human services could promulgate its own standards. While denying that administrative costs of the current multiple-payer system are $100 billion per year, the then-Secretary of HHS estimated that these new systems would save $24 billion per year.

Comment. Conservative observers endorsed the Bush/Chafee plan because they believe in altering the present insurance market system to expand access and strengthen consumer power, but retaining its basic structure.

Critics of this approach, however, said it advocated getting more people into managed care without providing a way to do it. They also criticized the subsidy to purchase insurance ($3,750 for a moderate-income family of three) as inadequate,and the lack of a proposal for financing the plan's startup.

1-C. House Republican Program
       (introduced by 89 House Republicans, June 4, 1992)

To increase access. The House Republican program proposes to set up accounts called Medisave. Derived from employer and employee tax-deductible contributions, these accounts would serve to purchase health insurance. All health and long-term care expenditures from these accounts would be tax-free.

Employers with up to 100 workers could form groups for purchasing health insurance with community-rated premiums. Insurers would have to offer small employers both a basic plan for essential health benefits, and a standard plan, comparable to coverage now generally available. Employees could not be disqualified by pre-existing conditions, nor could they be locked-in, that is lose coverage by job change.

The House Republican would also raise to 100% the current 25% deduction allowed to the self-employed for medical expenses, and increase funding for community and migrant health centers.

Cost containment. This program standardizes claims processing and requires hospitals to establish an electronic patient-care information system by January 1, 1996. It would reform medical mal practice liability and prohibit physician self-referrals.

Mandated Employer Insurance Programs (play-or-pay)

Mandated employer insurance programs aim to achieve universal access to medical care by requiring that all employers provide medical insurance to their employees, and by establishing a government agency to insure all others. Some of these play-or-pay programs permit employers, instead of insuring their employees, to pay an equivalent tax to the government which, in turn, insures the employees through an alternative public program (such as, in some instances, Medicare).

Most often, the government agency, established under these programs would insure the self-employed, non-workers and the poor.

Mandating employer-funded health insurance alone would pro vide insurance for 24 million workers and dependents, or two-thirds of the presently uninsured. It was a play-or-pay type of program that the then-Governor Clinton and Senator Tsongas endorsed in their campaigns for the 1992 Democratic presidential nomination. Also, several of the Democratic Party's leading legislators introduced bills into the 1992 Congress based on the play-or-pay principle.

Proponents of the play-or-pay principle say that eight out of 10 people under age 65 already received health insurance through work, and that therefore extending coverage to the entire working population through employment-based private insurance would minimize disruption. Mandatory insurance is necessary, they say, because it spreads risk equally, rather than making the insured, or tax-payer, bear the hidden costs for the care of the uninsured. They also point out that including low-risk people in the plan keeps costs down for all, rather than making individuals at greater risk pay more. Finally, proponents point out that play-or-pay programs retain the employer-based private insurance system already in place and incorporate the cost-containment features of Medicare.

Critics of mandated employer insurance programs offer no means to control the rate of acceleration of medical-care costs. (From 1965 to 1989, business spending for health benefits rose from 2.2% to 8.3% of wages and salaries, and from 8.4% to 56.4% of pre-tax corporate profits.) They add that administrative expense could remain a serious cost, and that "job-lock" and experience-rated rather than community rating for premiums could continue.

Furthermore, critics say the play-or-pay programs could curb job opportunities for low-skilled workers by forcing employers to pay relatively high insurance costs for them, and employers would be encouraged to use part-timers because they do not have to provide them with health benefits. Also, many of these plans include only workers for large companies, do not adequately cover part-time workers and occasionally even overlook dependents. Employers, if prohibited from reducing benefits or coverage, would resort to increasingly tighter controls over the most basic health decisions of American families. And, since the unemployed would be in a government provided plan, there would be a tendency to discriminate against them, encouraging two-tiered care. The American Medical Association objects to pay-or-play plans on the grounds that most employers would likely opt for the cheaper "pay option", unfairly forcing providers to negotiate with a single payer.

In reaction to some of these criticism, the Democratic Congressional delegation in June 1992 made a number of additions to their program proposals. They said that the government should increase regulation of health insurance to assure wider access to people with past health problems and to prevent "job-lock", and should allow the self-employed to deduct 100% of health insurance expenses after January 1, 1993. They also proposed establishing a national global budget for health expenditures and mandating negotiation for provider payments within this budget. Along with the Republicans, they endorsed tort and administrative reforms.

Then in late September 1992, candidate Clinton proposed that small employers band together to obtain community-rated premiums, and that they also receive tax-credits to help offset the cost of insuring their employees. He also supported the managed- competition concept.

2-A.   Universal Health Insurance, with Managed Competition and Managed Care

Alain Enthoven, a health economist teaching at Stanford University, and his colleagues have assembled over a period of years a program for universal health insurance, with managed competition and managed care. Their contribution is influential, and its various parts serve as paradigms for similar programs proposed by others. Enthoven's concept of "managed competition" has partly inspired recent British NHS reforms. Even President Bush, in August 1992, endorsed the managed-competition concept. Supported and propelled by the influential Jackson Hole Group, Enthoven's program will likely be the basis for the Clinton administration's medical care reform program.

To increase access. Enthoven recommends large employers, or sponsors, would be required to offer full-time employees a choice of "qualified plans" (see definition below) and to pay 80% of the premium for the cheapest such plan. The employer, who currently can deduct from his taxes 100% of employees' health benefits, could deduct only this 80%. Employees would pay the remaining 20%, and the added cost of any more elaborate plan that they choose. Employers would be required to pay to a public sponsor (see below) an eight percent payroll tax on the first $22,500 of the wages or salaries of all part-time or seasonal workers, unless these workers are otherwise provided with a health plan.

A qualified health plan would be any managed-care entity, such as HMOs or PPIs that met governmental defined standards, and provide a basic benefits package, called "basic health services". A qualified plan could not exclude coverage because of pre-existing conditions.

The federal government would require the states to set up a "public sponsor" to supply insurance for the self- employed, employees of small businesses and all those not otherwise covered, such as retirees under age 65. These individuals would pay their public sponsor, through the income tax system, eight percent of their adjusted gross income, up to an income ceiling related to their household size. The public sponsor would contribute a fixed amount equal to 80% of the cost of the average plan that meets minimum federal standards. The enrollee (in addition to the eight percent) would pay 20% of the cost. Enthoven and his colleagues believe the 80% level is low enough for efficient plans to compete with inefficient plans for subscribers, and high enough to attract healthy persons who think they won't need insurance to nevertheless subscribe. (Others call Enthoven's public sponsors: "Health Insurance Purchasing Cooperatives (HIPCs)", or "Purchasing Alliances".)

Under the Enthoven program the federal government would subsidize the premium payments of poor families. The government would subsidize the entire basic health plan premium payment for families whose income falls below the poverty level ($13,400 for a family of four in 1992). For families with an income between 100% and 150% of the poverty level, the subsidy would decrease to zero as the income approached 150% of poverty level. The subsidy would be available both to full time employees and to those covered by the public sponsor.

Employers with fewer than 25 full-time employees could buy basic coverage for their employees through the public sponsor. They thus would realize the savings from community-rated premiums now available only to large groups, and would not be required to pay more than 8% of their total payroll for this coverage. If the small business employers' required 80% contribution for basic health insurance exceeded eight percent of payroll, the public sponsor would subsidize the necessary amount beyond eight percent.

Financing. Under the Enthoven program, the government would collect from three sources: (1) the payroll tax paid by employers for other than full-time workers; (2) taxes from self- employed persons and others eligible to buy insurance from a public sponsor; and (3) taxes employees pay on employers' contributions beyond the amount they're allowed to exclude from their taxable income. (Those contributions are currently 100% excludable, and employers can also deduct them as a business expense.)

The federal government would need the revenue from the above three sources to replace money lost from the reduction in taxable wages when employers deduct contributions to the health insurance premiums of previously uninsured workers. The states will also need revenues to support their public sponsor agencies, which will: (1) subsidize 80% of the cost of an average health plan for households in which no member is a full-time worker; (2) subsidize some small businesses (those whose non-subsidized costs exceed eight percent of payroll) for coverage through the public sponsor; (3) subsidize an individual's share of the premium when the family income is less than 150% of the poverty level; and 4) cover the increased cost to the Federal Employee's Health Benefits Program.

The Enthoven program envisions the federal and state governments sharing subsidy costs. For example, the federal government would pay the public sponsor one-half the cost of the premium cost of a basic medical-care plan for each enrollee. The states would pay up to 30% of their public sponsors' costs (which includes 80% of each enrollee's premium), varying according to regional medical care costs. Medicaid and Medicare programs could continue, but the public sponsors might assist these programs. For instance, Medicaid might contract through the public sponsor to provide coverage for families on welfare, in order to ease the transition from welfare to work when, and if, this should occur. Medicare might use the public sponsors as brokers for HMO enrollment of its beneficiaries.

The cost to state governments of providing the 30% subsidy for individuals obligated to buy insurance directly from their public sponsor, will be about $5.2 billion. However, this would be offset by savings from no longer needing to pay for the medical care of their uninsured poor.

Proponents believe that the Enthoven program would be federally budget-neutral: since the estimated $12.8 billion) needed for the program would be balanced by increased tax revenues. After its first year of operation, proponents estimate it would decrease national expenditures by about $15 billion per year.

Cost containment. Through managed competition the Enthoven program would have large companies or state agencies, called sponsors, contract with health plans competing for their employees or enrollees. Each sponsor would monitor the medical-care market, creating what Enthoven calls "a process of informed, cost- conscious consumer choice that would offer the reward of more subscribers to health plans whose providers delivered high- quality care economically." Because these sponsors - either large employers or public agencies - would have the resources to be well-informed and control enough patients to be a potent competitive force, they would be able to act intelligently in the marketplace, correcting the market flaw caused by uninformed, unmotivated or weak individuals or companies. This is the basic concept of managed competition.

Enthoven believes managed competition will inspire outcome-of-treatment research and audits of provider efficiency, both of which is now seriously lacking.

The sponsors would have to offer their enrollees a variety of "qualified health plans". Since only 80% of the premium contributed by the employer would be tax deductible to the employee, the employee would be encouraged to seek out the least expensive plan. The more expensive the plan above his required 20% contribution for the basic plan, the more he would have to pay with his own non-tax-deductible dollars. Since managed-care plans (HMOs or PPOs) are cheaper than fee-for-service medical care, they would be favored.

Managed-care plans would compete to obtain contracts from sponsors and appeal to patients. Such plans would have incentive to give good value for money despite their incentive to control expenditures. At the same time, doctors and hospitals would be forced to join plans, or form new HMOs or PPOs, that would offer competitive prices and services.

Macro-rationing - The Enthoven program would allow only a certain amount of health insurance costs to be deducted from taxes, thus giving employers incentive to pick the cheapest plan that provides basic medical-care coverage.

Micro-rationing - Since only a portion of health costs would be tax-deductible, subscribers would be attracted to lower costs plans that would supply less options for care. Under managed care, providers freed from the profit incentive would use technology assessment and outcome records to offer patients only care that is effective. Management audits would prevent doctors from conserving treatment over-zealously in response to their "reversed" economic incentive - the less they spend, the more money remains for themselves.

Comment. Under the Enthoven program, 22 million of the currently estimated 35 million uninsured Americans would be covered by their employers. The remaining 13 million would be eligible to purchase subsidized coverage from a public sponsor. Critics believe as much as $80 billion per year in taxes would be required to insure the poor.

This is a consumer-choice program, because it offers a choice among health plans and an opportunity to exercise cost-quality judgments reflecting consumer preferences. Since they would compete both for subscribers and for physician participation, these health plans would be both responsive to patients and respectful of doctors' professional judgments and aspirations.

The Enthoven program would not be a radical change from the present system. It would not cause a major change in the coverage of most employed people. However, competition for contracts would lead to vertical integration of services (see glossary).

Enthoven and colleagues admitted that, if starting from scratch, they would not choose an employment-based system, but the existence of $200 billion of vested retirement interest and employer liabilities can't be ignored.

Since the Enthoven program reforms the entire medical-care system, its provision of insurance for everyone should not be inflationary. The program gives patients and providers incentives to conserve costs and, since there is already an adequate supply of physicians and hospital facilities, increasing the numbers of insured would not bid up prices substantially.

While small businesses will complain of the added costs, Enthoven believes the current system is worse, allowing employers and employees who don't participate in health insurance, but receive care, to take a "free ride" at the expense of other employers and taxpayers.

These planners believe their program gives doctors the necessary economic and professional incentives to make the plan in which they participate succeed. These doctors, working in concert with their plan administrators who have similar incentives, will have to provide good care in order to compete for patients, and will have to conserve expenditures in order to maximize the pool from which their incomes would be derived. Doctors probably would be paid on a performance-based system, at a level somewhere between fee-for-service and salaries, using peer judgment and various performance indicators.

This managed-competition program would have some negative effects on employment, particularly of the young and unskilled. It would in effect raise the minimum wage by eight percent, the amount small employers or larger employers of part-time help would have to contribute to the public sponsor for each worker.

Critics of this program also point to the length of time it would take to accomplish its goals, since it requires a fundamental restructuring of the American health system. They also object because managed-competition, to function, requires a critical mass of 200,000 to 500,000 of health consumers in any one area as well as convenient access to health facilities, and one-third of Americans live in less populated areas and far from a doctor or hospital. Indeed, one-half of all Americans live in areas that cannot support more than one large managed-care organization, making dependence on competition to control the American medical-care system overly optimistic.

Others object that the Enthoven program would lock patients and doctors into plans managed by insurance companies. They say it would deprive consumers and health providers of choice, and granting the insurance industry even greater power than it has in the current system. Ultimately, they say, patients would be herded into a limited number of huge HMOs that manage salaried physicians. This would create a tiered system of care, with poorer people in cut-rate HMOs and the more affluent able to afford plans with more and better benefits.

A number of prominent politicians and planners forming the "Jackson Hole Group" endorsed the Enthoven program. in August 1992, Senators David Durenberger (R-MN) and Jeff Bingaman (D-NM), both Jackson Hole members, introduced legislation, the Health Insurance Purchasing Cooperatives Act (S. 3165), to provide states with "seed money" to organize consortia to provide health insurance for employees of firms with 50 or fewer workers, as a step towards a nation-wide managed-competition, managed-care program. The proposed legislation also provided for uniform electronic billing and other administrative reforms.

John Garamendi, California's Insurance Commissioner, in February 1992 proposed a program for California essentially similar to the one first proposed by Enthoven but including global budgeting.

The Emeritus Editor of The New England Journal of Medicine, Arnold Relman, has endorsed The Enthoven program, but stresses that physicians should maintain their independence when practicing in groups, rather than be disciplined by managers. More precisely, he advocates physician-sponsored and directed HMOs, with peer-directed, as well as economic, incentives to conserve resources. He has also advocated a single-payer, Canadian-style system of universal government insurance, but with HMOs providing medical care, and with physicians on salary in order to remove the economic incentive for them to unduly conserve the amount of medical care they offer.

A group of large businesses, consumer groups and associations of medical-care providers calling themselves "National Leadership Coalition for Health Care Reform" endorsed the Enthoven program in a New England Journal of Medicine article of November 19, 1992. They suggested adding as cost containment features separate prospective budgets for operating and capital expenses, with limitations on provider payments. They also recommended the development of practice guidelines based on outcomes research, as well as provisions for simplified administration, and tort reform.

In December 1992, the Health Insurance Association of America, capitulating to the inevitability of change, agreed to managed competition by calling for a new federal law. That law would require coverage for all Americans, limit tax credit to the cost of a defined set of basic benefits, and prevent state-imposed barriers to managed care. The insurers viewed managed competition as creating a large new market for them, but one in which competition for new subscribers would hold down premium costs.

2-B. *Pepper Commission Program (U.S. Bipartisan Commission on Comprehensive Health Care)*

The Pepper Commission, consisting of six members from each part of Congress and three presidential appointees, concluded in May 1991 that national health insurance is not politically feasible, because shifting so many dollars from the private to the public sector would be too disruptive. On the other hand, patching up the present system with more incremental changes would not achieve universal access to medical care. Therefore the Pepper Commission proposed the "Health Care Access and Reform Act of 1991".

To increase access. Employers with more than 100 employees must insure all workers and their families.

Smaller employers would have access to insurance for their employees by reform of the private insurance industry. Insurers of small businesses would be encouraged to pool their risks by re-insurance, to facilitate their offering community-based premium rates. To ease the costs of this insurance, the premiums for unincorporated businesses and the self-employed would be 100% tax-deductible, as they are now for incorporated businesses. For 5 years, employers of less than 25 workers and a payroll of less than $18,000 per worker would receive a governmental subsidy of 40% of their premium costs.

The Pepper Commission also recommended setting up a new federal program to be administered as part of, or in conjunction with, Medicare. Covering non-workers and the self-employed, and replacing Medicaid for the poor, this program would pay providers by the same rules and rates as Medicare. The minimum benefit package would provide both primary and catastrophic care and would emphasize preventive care services.

Employers would be allowed to choose between purchasing insurance privately or from the newly established federal program. The price for public coverage, if this was to be chosen, would be five to eight percent of the payroll, putting a cap on employers' obligations and avoiding excessive costs for part-time workers.

Financing. The Commission estimated that implementing their recommendations to achieve universal access would cost less than two percent more than the present system which, in 1990, would have been $12 billion. Fifty percent of this in crease would go to hospitals, 25% to doctors and the rest to other professionals and services.

The Pepper Commission recommended several shifts in supporting medical-care costs. The federal government would share with employers the costs of insurance premiums saving companies who now insure their employees $13 billion, and individuals and families $19 billion. Medicaid costs would be limited to past levels, saving state and local governments $7 billion. But employers who hadn't previously provided worker health insurance would now have to pay $28 billion - an average of four percent of after-tax payroll, but as high as seven percent for any single employer. New federal expenditures would be $24 billion, which would have to come from new taxes.

Cost containment. *Macro-rationing* - the Medicare approach, prospective payments to hospital (DRGs) and resource-based relative value scale payments for physicians (RBRVSs), would apply to all newly-included recipients. To help consumers and insurers become more prudent purchasers of medical care, the Commission recommended the federal government collect and publish information on the outcome of treatments, development of practice guidelines, quality assurance studies, and similar matters.

Micro-rationing - The Pepper Commission recommended consumers share up to 20% of the premium, and deductibles up to $250 per person and $500 per family, according to ability to pay. However, no individual or family should pay more than $3000 annually for premium and deductibles combined, and people with incomes below 100% of the federal poverty level would pay neither premiums nor copayments. Subsidies on a sliding scale would be available for persons with incomes up to twice the poverty level. In addition, private insurers and employers would offer monetary incentives to join HMOs and PPOs.

The Commission left remedies for the problems and costs of malpractice for further study.

Comment. Critics said that despite Commission estimates, the Pepper Commission plan would add $66.2 billion to medical-care costs for two reasons. The first was that its cost containment measures for the newly covered were limited to only those provided by Medicare.

Secondly, while more people than previously would go on Medicare, large segments of the population would remain out of Medicare, and unaffected by its cost containment measures.

The Pepper Commission proposals differ from Enthoven's program in two respects. First, the government health insurance agency would be national, rather than state-sponsored. Second, the Pepper recommendations do not concentrate on promoting competition in the delivery of medical care.

2-C. HealthAmerica: Affordable Health Care for All Americans Act (bill S 1227, sponsored by Sen. George Mitchell (D, Maine) introduced June 1991, and amended January 1992)

To increase access. Like the Pepper Commission, the Mitchell bill requires each employer to insure each employee and family. However, it permits even large employers to chose to make an equal contribution to the national government's insurance program, to be called AmeriCare. The Mitchell bill also defines an employee as anyone who normally performs one or more hours per week for a specific employer. Small businesses that can't afford coverage would receive a tax credit for up to 25% of the cost of a qualified group health plan. Self-employed individuals without employees could deduct from their taxes the lowest cost of a qualified plan, or the cost of enrollment in the federal insurance program, whichever is less. Business owner-operators could deduct the cost of their own health insurance premiums up to the cost of the premium paid on behalf of their employees. However, that deduction could not exceed the taxable income from the business.

HealthAmerica would established state consortia (Americares) managed by boards of insurers, providers and consumers, and supported initially by federal grants. Each consortium would have to enroll all small-share health insurance companies as members. The consortia would establish a claim payment fund, capitalized by public and private contributions and enrollee assessments reflecting the amount paid on behalf of each enrollee.

AmeriCare would provide the same basic benefits as would be provided by private employment plans, and would reimburse at the same amounts and conditions as Medicare. Families with below poverty-level incomes would not have to pay premiums, copayments or deductibles. Near-poverty families (with income below 200% of poverty level) would pay an indexed monthly rate, not to exceed 3% of family income. Families from 200% to 400% above the poverty level would make indexed contributions ranging from 3.5% to 5% of annual family income.

AmeriCare which would take over the acute care portion of Medicaid would be administered by the states. Each state would establish an agency, other than the Medicaid agency, to administer AmeriCare. It would provide basic benefits of the program to any pregnant woman or child not otherwise covered by a non-governmental program, to any employee or family member for whom an employer makes a contribution under this "play-or-pay" bill, and to any individual not otherwise covered.

Each state would provide a number of managed-care plans for individuals to choose from, with yearly options to change. Physicians would receive incentives that would comply, at minimum, with Medicare's quality guidelines. There would also be a system of rate assessment that would minimize risk- segmentation of beneficiaries or "cherry-picking".

Each state would set up "Quality Improvement Boards" to review the quality of medical care provided and establish mechanisms to encourage continuous improvement. Each board would include seven medical-care providers, four insurers and purchasers, and four medical-care researchers and consumers. These boards would certify providers, and be able to deny certification if a provider's service did not conform to established guidelines.

Financing. Employers would pay premiums for their own plans or for enrolling their employees in AmeriCare. Other enrollees in AmeriCare would pay their own premiums. Some enrollees would also pay their own cost-sharing contributions.

But estimates are that AmeriCare would require $5 billion in new taxes the first year, and $11 billion by the fifth year when it would be fully operational.

Cost containment. *Macro-rationing* - An independent agency, the "Federal Health Expenditure Board" would be established to utilize the single-payer concept. This board would develop national standards for affordable health expenditures, access and quality, convene and oversee negotiations between providers and purchasers to develop payment rates, and recommend payment levels and other cost-containment measures, such as increased utilization of managed care, alternatives to institutionalization, and procedures for allocation and limitation of capital investment. The board would also establish uniform billing and claim forms, and recommend rates, budgets and other measures to help meet expenditure goals while assuring access to quality and affordable care under federal health insurance programs. If negotiators fail to agree on payment rates or any other matter, the Board is to issue binding rates or directives.

In addition, the state consortia would develop procedures for allocating capital among providers to encourage rational distribution of medical-care providers. And, if they so desired, states could adopt single-payer insurance programs, like the Canadian system, rather than the play-or-pay approach.

Micro-rationing - The Federal Health Expenditure Board through its rate setting power, aided by the power of the state agencies to allocate funds, would foster development of managed-care plans. Peer Review Organizations (PROs) would monitor the quality and cost-effectiveness of care in AmeriCare plans. Utilization review procedures for assessing doctors and controlling their excess treatments would be enhanced by a funding increase of $50,000,000 to expand the activities of the Agency for Health Care Policy and Research in outcomes research and technology assessment, and in developing treatment guide lines.

Fully employed individuals would pay 20% of the monthly premium. Deductible and co-pay rules would remain the same as Medicare and be extended to those insured by AmeriCare.

The Federal Health Expenditure Board would encourage managed competition by requiring reports on the quality and cost of care of individual providers. The Board then would issue reports on each provider at least annually, to assist purchasers in evaluating providers.

In addition, grants would be awarded to develop, demonstrate and evaluate innovative methods for reducing medical-care costs. States could obtain grants to develop and implement malpractice reforms.

Comment. The HealthAmerica program includes many features of Enthoven's proposal, with less emphasis on managed competition. In addition, it includes cost-control by government prospective global budgeting - similar to nationalized systems abroad - with negotiations between insurers, providers and consumers determining division of the budgeted amount. (Similar to state-mandated insurance systems in other countries.)

Republican-funded studies estimate that this program and others like it would add $36 billion to federal Medicaid costs. If such a program had been in effect in 1989, say those studies, businesses would have paid an additional $28 billion for medical care, while costs to small employers would have risen 71%, or $11 billion. However,these costs would have been partially offset by the elimination of uncompensated care, for which employers had been forced to pay partially.

While HealthAmerica makes no provision for long-term care, another bill introduced by Sen. Mitchell in April 1992 would provide disabled individuals up to 88 hours per month of services including home nursing care, adult day care, and personal assistance, as well as two six months episodes of nursing home care. The estimated cost of this disabled care is $45 billion annually.

Mitchell conceded that the cost of these acute and long-term care programs would prevent these bills' passage in the near future.

While Senators Rockefeller, Kennedy, and Riegle endorsed the Mitchell bill, Rep. Dan Rostenkowski (D-Ill) proposed a similar program (HR 3205, Health Insurance and Cost Control Act of 1991), with several differences.First, the Rostenkowski bill enhanced Medicare benefits and expanded them to apply to ages 60-64. His program would be financed by a nine percent income surtax, an increase in Medicare payroll tax, and Medicare tax wage base increase to $200,000. His cost containment measures would not include malpractice reform, managed care or practice guidelines from outcomes research, but would include following all current Medicare payment rules. The American College of Surgeons protested this latter proposal because Medicare physician payment rates, by 1992, averaged about 35% less than those of private insurers.

2-D.   *Health Reform Bill of 1992 sponsored by Congressmen Richard Gephardt (D-Mo) and Pete Stark (D-Cal) (introduced June 1992)*

To increase access. A play-or-pay program, the Gephardt-Stark bill requires employers to provide insurance or pay a tax for workers to be covered by a governmental agency.

Self-employed workers' health insurance premiums would be 100% tax-deductible beginning 1994 (replacing the previous 25% deduction).

All health insurance premiums would be community-rated, and insurers would be forbidden to discriminate be cause of previous health record or any other factor.

Medicaid eligibility would be expanded to include all with incomes below 125% of the poverty level by 2001, and below 133% in 2002; all pregnant women and children to age 6 in families with incomes below 200% of poverty level as of 1998; and, by 1999, children through age 18 from families with incomes below 200% of the poverty level.

The Gephardt-Stark program would create a Federal Health Insurance Program for Children, covering children through age 18 with rules and benefits similar to Medicare's. This program would be available regardless of income. Employers (except those already providing coverage as of 1/1/92) or parents would pay premiums, estimated at $1300 per year. Out-of-pocket expenses would be limited to $3000 annually.

The Gephardt-Stark program would add several benefits not included in Medicare, such as annual mammograms for women over 65, colon-rectal screening, tetanus and influenza vaccinations and, in 1996, prescription drug costs with an $800 deductible rising to $900 in 1998.

Financing. Using current Medicare payment methods (DRGs and RVRBSs) to set payment rates for various medical-care categories, and the Secretary of Health and Human Services would impose (or cap) mandatory reductions in growth of spending.

Cost containment. This bill would limit annual growth of health expenditures to six percent per year.

Medicare rules and caps would apply to all patients, and Medicare's doctor "self-referral" ban would be extended to other services and for all patients, even those not insured by Medicare.

This program also provides for administrative simplifications including electronic billing, uniform reporting on patient outcomes, and encourages managed care by permitting HMOs to opt out of the Medicare payment system.

2-E.   *Health-Access-America - The AMA Program*

To increase access. The AMA's proposed program can be dubbed, rather than play-or-pay, a play-or-else program. It requires employers, who would receive tax help, to pay for health insurance for all full-time employees. Large self-insured employers would have to participate in private, not-for-profit uninsured and uninsurable risk pools. The states would set up these pools, and would offer small businesses with fewer than 25 employees access to a basic benefits policy at large group rates. Their premiums paid for their employees would be 100% tax-deductible as would be those paid by the self-employed, and any others who have to pay their own insurance. Insurers would be forbidden to deny coverage for pre-existing conditions, or to anyone previously insured by a spouse's employers, or to anyone who has changed jobs.

Employers would also have to pay the medical bills of uninsured workers, plus a penalty - hence this program "play-or-else" label.

The AMA program would reform Medicaid to assure anyone below the poverty level access to medical care adequate for all their needs - including prescription drugs, rehabilitative and emergency services - regardless of state of residence. It would also expand Medicaid reimbursement levels to those of Medicare, so that providers won't deny services.

Health Access America would reform Medicare so as to protect continued access by senior citizens, even when the present tax contributions ratio of 4 workers to each single Medicare beneficiary drops to two to one, as is projected for 2050. This reform would also provide for catastrophic benefits to be funded through individual and employer tax contributions during the working years.

It would finance long-term care through expansion of private sector coverage, encouraged by tax-incentives, an asset protection program, and coverage for all those below the poverty level provided by Medicaid. Those with incomes between 100% and 200% of the poverty level would receive sliding scale subsidies for buying long-term care insurance. Employer-provided long-term care insurance would be tax-deductible, and a new tax credit would encourage families to give care to their own elderly or disabled members.

In addition, the AMA program would provide tax incentives for individual retirement, or health accounts. It would extend medical benefits to part-time workers with vouchers equal to a set percentage of gross pay.

Cost containment. *Micro-rationing* - The AMA program calls legislative appropriations for medical-care assessment research to support development of professional practice parameters. It acknowledges managed care as an alternative to the traditional pluralistic delivery system.

The AMA proposes managed competition through limiting the amount of employer-provided health insurance that is tax-exempt to the employee. Employees who chose health insurance plans with premiums less expensive than those chosen by their employers would receive tax-exempt rebates. (Such a measure would reward people for choosing medical-care insurance.)

Furthermore, the AMA program calls for repeal of the many "state-mandated-special-benefit laws" (see glossary), reform of professional liability laws, and for giving incentives to payers and providers to switch to uniform electronic billing.

Comment. The AMA's play-or-else program is somewhat similar to the Democratic Party's play-or-pay proposals, but it also incorporates the Republican Party approach of broadening private insurance coverage through tax credits for premiums for the more affluent and vouchers for the poor to buy private insurance.

2-F. State Mandated Employer Insurance Programs

Lawmakers in several states have already enacted new medical-care legislation to expand medical-care coverage to all employed people. And by 1993, in anticipation of President Clinton's commitment to managed competition, nine states had ready for enactment complementary programs setting up public sponsors and boards to license health plans and determine basic benefits packages. (See, for example, Florida's program detailed below.) These states hoped, readying their plans in anticipation of the new national program, would position them well to argue for flexibility in their own programs.

Hawaii

Since 1974, Hawaii has required employers to provide insurance for specified acute medical-care benefits to those employed more than 20 hours per week, including workers with health problems. As a result, 92% of Hawaiians have had health insurance compared to the national average of 84%. Employers must pay at least 50% of the premium; with employees paying up to 50%, but not more than 1.5% of wages. There are copayments for most services.

Employers are not required to cover their employees' dependents, but a large majority of employers do so voluntarily at no cost to the employee. The two major insurers for businesses with 100 or fewer employees, Blue Cross and Kaiser Permanente, have single risk pools, so even small businesses pay single, community-rated premiums. People not covered at work or by Medicaid or Medicare have had access since 1990 to a state subsidized medical program that provides care on a sliding scale basis for those with incomes below 300% of the poverty level. The poorest Hawaiians pay nothing for this program, others pay up to $60 per month for an individual and $140 for a family. This state program provides only for 12 physicians visits and 5 days of hospitalization per year. In 1989, prior to this program for the poor, 3.5% of the Hawaiian population remained uncovered by any kind of health insurance.

Seventy percent of Hawaiians receive their medical care through two insurers, Blue Cross/Blue Shield and Kaiser Permanente (an HMO). This relationship approximates a one-payer system insofar as these two insurers, with their large market shares, are able to exert considerable control over medical-care fees and charges.

Proponents of Hawaii's program point out that it consumes less resources than does medical care nationally: in 1992, 7.8% of gross Hawaiian product compared to 11.2% of GNP in the United States. Availability of early treatment for all and the ability to treat most ailments in physician's offices and not in expensive emergency room settings accounts for Hawaii's edge. It is claimed that Hawaii's health program illustrates that universal access is itself a powerful cost-containment technique.

However, critics of the Hawaiian program point out that Hawaii has a higher rate of employment and fewer poor people than other states as well as a healthier population. Further more, since it's in the center of the ocean, Hawaiian employers cannot move elsewhere to flee the mandated health insurance costs. Moreover, although Hawaiian health costs remain lower than on the mainland, their rate of escalation is the same.

Massachusetts

The Massachusetts Health Security Act was passed in 1988 to achieve universal coverage by 1992. It was to allow uninsured residents of the state to obtain health insurance in several different ways. Disabled adults wishing to work and disabled children of working parents were to obtain primary and supplemental insurance through a program known as Commonwealth by the end of 1988. All college students were to have health insurance either privately or through their schools by 1989. In 1990 businesses with 50 or fewer employees providing health insurance to their employees - without having offered it in the previous 3 years - were to obtain a two year tax-credit for 20% of the insurance premium the first year and for 10% for the second year.

The following year, in 1991, persons on relief were to be enrolled in prepaid health insurance plans, paid for with state appropriations. And in 1992 employers with six or more employees were to be required to contribute, for each employee working at least 20 hours per week in a permanent job, $1680 to a state-administered medical security trust fund. This fund was to have offered insurance to uninsured workers and workers receiving unemployment compensation. Employers who already offered health insurance to their employees could have deducted those expenditures from their required contributions. Thus, all Massachusetts residents who were without employer-sponsored health insurance were to be able to purchase health insurance from the Department of Medical Security by 1992. However, implementation of this law has been delayed until 1995.

Comment. This state law was passed because employers were overwhelmed by the rising cost of health insurance premiums contributed to by the shifting of the costs of uncompensated hospital care for those uninsured to the insured. Those believing Massachusetts needed universal coverage battled others concerned that achieving this goal would hurt small employers. The enacted Law was a compromise providing all residents the opportunity to buy a health insurance policy more cheaply than previously. However, the compromise law required only employers with six or more employees to provide insurance. Since, in addition, the law did not apply to employees working less than 20 hours, or temporarily or seasonally, it was estimated that the Bill would provide insurance for only 43% of the uninsured and only 55% of the working uninsured. Those not covered would have to purchase the reduced rate policies, and most, but not all, said they would be willing.

Interestingly, contrary to the impression of most, the uninsured in Massachusetts were not persons below the poverty level. Sixty-six percent of the eight percent who were uninsured were in households with an income above the poverty level; 84% of the uninsured lived in a household with an employed adult, usually by a small or medium-sized business. Most uninsured adults said that they had no insurance because of its cost, due to pre-existing medical conditions, or because they had not worked enough hours to be eligible for employer-provided insurance.

But by the middle of 1992, depressed business conditions and the fiscal state crisis made repeal of the Massachusetts Health Security Act, or a delay in its meaningful implementation, seem very likely. Still, most state residents - 56% in 1991, down from 64% in 1990 - who knew of the law were still in favor of it. Interestingly, in 1991 28% of those polled had never heard of the law, including 41% of the uninsured and 56% of the poor.

Florida

In March 1992, Florida enacted a program similar to the Massachusetts plan for the uninsured. There are 2.5 million uninsured in Florida in a total population of 13 million, and the law is scheduled to take effect in 1995. Employers will have the option of providing basic medical-care insurance for their workers, with tax incentives to use managed-care plans, or be taxed to finance coverage.

In April 1993, a managed-competition program was enacted in Florida. It created eleven Community Health Purchasing Alliances, which are pools of employers, government workers and the poor. They will bargain with insurers and providers for the lowest rates. The insurers will offer community-rated premiums and the Alliances will determine the medical-care plans to be offered. However, the law did not specify how the cost of the program - especially to insure the presently uninsured - was to be met, nor the plan's minimum benefits, nor treatment guide lines for participating doctors.

Minnesota

In April 1992, the Minnesota legislature established MinnesotaCare (formerly called HealthRight) to provide state-subsidized insurance to some of its 370,000 uninsured residents. At that time, 92% of the state's 4.4 million people were insured. Of the uninsured, an estimated 158,000 were self-employed, or worked for small businesses and were not eligible for Medicaid, but, earning less than $38,300, they could not afford health insurance. The bill extended basic coverage to these self-employed or small-business employees, charging them amounts ranging from 1.5% of income for the poorest to 10% for those relatively well off. That meant a family of three earning $10,000 a year paid $12.53 per month, and a family with a yearly income of $28,000 paid $300 a month. The state subsidized the rest of the premium. The law also prohibits experience-rating insurance premiums. Basic coverage includes outpatient services, dental services, and prescriptions. Some services require copayments, for example, $25 for eyeglasses. Limited inpatient services, up to $10,000 per year, were added July 1, 1993.

Expected to cost $250 million a year, MinnesotaCare is financed by an added 5% tax on cigarettes and a 2% tax on gross revenue of medical-care providers, including hospitals, doctors, and dentists. Starting in 1996, there will be a 1% tax on HMOs and health service organizations such as Blue Cross and Blue Shield.

The state also created a Health Care Cost Containment Commission for the purpose of macro-rationing. It will set state targets for reducing the annual rise in medical-care costs, and provide for state review of medical technology costing more than $500,000 before granting permission to purchase. Stringent restrictions were imposed on doctor referral to medical facilities in which they have an interest.

2-G.   *Play-or-Pay Medicaid or Medicare Proposals*

Both the *Kansas Employer Coalition on Health, Inc. Program* and the *Urban Institute Program* are permutations of the play-or-pay plan. They propose retention of Medicare, and merging Medicaid into a public plan set up to cover workers whose employers opt to pay a tax rather than self-insure, and for other individuals who buy into it. The public plan would insure the poor not eligible for Medicaid. They also propose federal takeover of long-term care from Medicaid to relieve states of this burden. Although both plans include a number of cost containment features such as governmental control of yearly rate increases, both would require raising taxes.

Pay-or-Play Medicare Program, proposed by Karen Davis, Johns Hopkins University would make the U.S. Medicare Program the government vehicle for carrying out the "pay" portion complementing employers' mandatory "play" through private insurance. The cost to employers would not exceed six percent of workers' wages, with employees responsible for the rest of their premiums, except if employers opted for Medicare. Then employees would have to contribute two percent of their earned income toward their Medicare coverage. The premiums of low-wage earners would be off-set by a credit on their earned income tax.

This Pay-or-Play Medicare program would give states the option of bringing all current Medicaid beneficiaries and others below the poverty income level into Medicare. Long-term care would remain under Medicaid. The remaining uninsured non-poor, estimated at five to eight million people, would automatically be covered by Medicare, and would be taxed 2% of their income as their premium.

Medicare cost sharing would be expanded to a deductible of $250 per person and $500 per family. A 20% co-insurance would apply to all services other than hospital care. Cost sharing would be limited to $1500 per individual or $3000 per family annually. Employers would be permitted to provide financial incentives for enrollment in managed-care plans.

Professor Davis estimates her proposal would cost the federal government about $25 billion per year. This program differs from the Pepper Commission's and other public-private plans because it does not stress reform of the private insurance market, such as requiring community rating, prohibiting exclusion of pre-existing conditions, or establishing risk-sharing pools. Instead, this proposal gives all employers and non-working individuals the option of Medicare coverage, with its administrative efficiency and cost-containment provisions. Private insurers would have the incentive of not losing enrollees to Medicare to improve their benefits at a competitive cost. "Dumping" of poor risks onto Medicare would be prevented by requiring employers to cover all employees under Medicare, or none. However, early retirees with health problems and without retiree benefits would find Medicare attractive.

Universal National Health Insurance Programs (Canadian-style)

Universal National Health Insurance Programs are single, comprehensive public insurance programs guaranteeing access to care for all. They are supported by taxation on businesses and individuals, have no copayments or deductibles, and allow free choice of provider. These programs are also called single-payer programs.

Many analysts believe that simply replacing the myriad of private insurers, Medicaid and Medicare with a single-payer mechanism would save enough money to pay for the expanded access provided by Canadian-style programs. Moreover, the macro-rationing techniques of a single-payer system and the prospective global budgeting that often accompany one another are long-term mechanisms for controlling escalation of costs. However, micro-rationing - as practiced by Canadian doctors and effected by queuing - would also be required to ensure the efficacy of these macro-rationing methods.

One estimate of the administrative savings of switching to a Canadian-like system was $55 billion for the year 1991, which would have paid for the estimated $48.2 billion cost to cover the 35 million uninsured that year. It is also estimated that the U.S. uninsured did use $36 billion of the $567 billion spent on health that year. This $36 million paid for "free care" in subsidized public hospitals, uncompensated care at private facilities shifted to the insured revenues and out-of-pocket services. Thus the claim that such savings would provide sufficient billions to pay for start-up costs of a comparable program for the United States.

Universal national health insurance programs differ from employer-based programs like those of the Pepper Commission, Enthoven, and the senate Democratic Leadership because they are financed through taxes, not by private premium payments. Some analysts favor tax financing because it makes cost containment depend upon changing the financial incentives for health plans and providers through a unified one payer reimbursement system, rather than relying on increasing cost-consciousness among health service users and individual health plan buyers. Tax financing also saves administrative expenses by preventing interruption of insurance for employees who change jobs.

Tax financing frees employers from administrative expense, particularly unaffordable to small firms, and eliminates a source of labor-management conflict. Employers are freed from providing health benefits for retirees; their health costs would be limited to a percentage of their payroll. This is particularly helpful to small businesses and those dependent on low-wage, part-time or temporary workers. Universal national health insurance also enlarges workers' choice of plans rather than limiting them to their employers' choices. And its unitary financing system avoids separating low-income groups off into Medicaid which then takes on a stigma of poor, underserved and likely to suffer from governmental budget cutting.

Critics of national health insurance say it increases government bureaucracy, and makes it possible for the government to dictate treatment decisions to doctors and hospitals. As practiced in Canada, it also forces people to queue for some non-emergency studies and treatments. Finally, many believe that national health insurance is not politically feasible, since it calls for such sweeping change, and even though it would ultimately cost less, it would initially require a tax increase of as much as $200 billion. In addition, a large number of forces - insurers, provider groups, health-care workers' unions, and others - are ranged against such a system.

3-A.   American College of Physician's Position

In 1990, the American College of Physicians published a position paper outlining the problems with the current medical-care system and certain conclusions varying with those reached by the AMA. The position of the prestigious College and several other doctors' groups demonstrates that American physicians are not united in the conservative approach to medical-care reform usually attributed to them.

In essence, the 1990 position paper of The American College of Physicians called for a nationwide program to assure medical care insurance coverage for all Americans. The College's committee noted that, in contrast to private insurance, publicly-funded programs don't include costs for profits, marketing, or premium collection. Overhead for the Canadian universal public health insurance system averages 2.5% of program costs, and overhead costs of Medicare and Medicaid amounted to less than 3% in 1983 and were closer to 2% of much larger total costs in 1990. Each one-percentage point reduction - achieved through administrative streamlining and correction of other inefficiencies - in the proportion of GNP used for medical care would yield savings of almost $60 billion per year. Although the position paper did not explicitly say so, its conclusion implied that a Canadian-style, single-payer public insurance program would save enough money from the present private insurance multiple payer system (whose overhead is more than 20%) to pay for insurance for the estimated 35 million presently without it.

However, in September 1992, the College modified its position, calling instead for a play-or-pay approach with a single-payer cost-containment mechanism and incremental changes to address problems such as tort reform and making insurance coverage more comprehensive. The revised program called for consolidating Medicare, Medicaid and other publicly financed health programs into a single public agency. This agency would insure all Americans not belonging to private plans, and allow them to join the insurance plan or managed-care program of their choice. Employers would be required to insure their employees, paying either a minimum 50% of the premium or paying a tax to the publicly financed program. Employers would not have to cover employees over age 60 or retirees, nor be responsible for catastrophic costs over $50,000 because the public program would assume those responsibilities.

The College also called for a national commission to place a cap on medical-care spending, to require private and public insurers to offer a uniform set of benefits covering "all medically effective and appropriate care", and to regulate the supply of doctors and hospitals. Rather than calling for managed competition, the College said this commission should limit doctor and hospital fees through negotiations with the states.

3-B.   Physicians-for-a-National-Health-Program (NHP) (1991)

To increase access. Through a Canadian-style single-payer, government financed national health insurance for everyone.

This NHP program would provide long-term care services, including medical, dental and nursing care, drugs and medical devices, and preventive services to supplement and be integrated with acute care services.

Financing. Payroll taxes would remain pegged at the amount employers and employees currently pay for group insurance. This amount represents at present 31% of total personal health expenditures in the United States.

Social Security payments for Medicare would likewise be pegged at present levels.

However, to make the payroll tax less regressive, the present Social Security cap would be removed so that higher earners would pay more and the employer's share of social security payments be reduced for small businesses.

The NHP would take the $157 billion in non-Social Security general government revenues for health that come from federal, state and local government levels and use it to finance 26% of the planned program. Since the current 31% of medical-care costs paid by individuals is the most regressive feature of current health funding, the NHP would replace these individual payments with a number of so-called "healthy revenues". These would include a new federal income tax bracket of 38% for families with incomes higher than $170,000; a cap on mortgage interest deductions for luxury homes; a 0.5% securities transfer tax; an increased energy tax; a tax increase on cigarettes to 32 cents per pack; a tax increase on alcohol to 25 cents per ounce; an excise tax on sources of water and air pollutants; and a tax on fossil fuels. These taxes would yield $124 billion per year, or 21% of the proposed NHP budget. Individuals would pay for the remaining 15% of NHP out-of-pocket.

Current for-profit providers would receive a fixed return on existing equity, setting up new for-profits would be forbidden.

Cost containment. *Macro-rationing* - State agencies would become the single payer for negotiating prospective budgets for institutions and fee schedules for payment to individual providers. Each state's operating budget for long-term care would be allocated to local LTC agencies. Institutional providers such as community agencies, nursing homes, home care agencies or social service organizations would negotiate a global operating budget with the local LTC agency. Alternatively, institutional providers could contract to provide integrated acute and LTC services on a per-capita basis. The state LTC agency would set explicit health planning goals, and capital expansion, separated from operating budgets, would be allocated according to these goals.

Micro-rationing - Each state would set up a long-term care system (LTC) with a Planning and Paying Board and a network of local LTC agencies to evaluate eligibility and needs, and to assign case managers.

Administrative expenses would be reduced.

Comments. The Physicians for a NHP deplore the current attempts of multiple payers in the United States to contain costs by micro-managing doctors through intrusive patient-by-patient utilization review as interference with the clinical freedom of doctors. They point out that macro-management by a single payer and macro-rationing through global budgets, on the other hand, enhances clinical freedom.

The NHP would not result in queuing, as in Canada, since its stated goal is not to lower the percentage of GNP consumed by American medical care, only to contain its rapid escalation. Since the United States spends a larger portion of GNP on medical care than does Canada, and this plan calls for enhancing the system through management, it would not cause queuing.

The Physicians for a NHP criticized employer-mandated insurance proposals, like the Pepper Commission's plan or the AMA's Health-Access-America plan, for having no cost control mechanisms, offering no improvement in coverage of those currently insured, and effecting no decrease in administrative costs. These plans, said the Physicians for a NHP would inevitably inflate costs, by extending coverage of those presently uninsured without offsetting expenditure reductions.

The sponsors of this Canadian-like proposal do not believe Enthoven's program with its competing managed-care insurers and higher patient copayments would hold costs in check. "Does forcing consumers to bear premium costs for higher-priced plans hold down over-all costs," they ask "or simply segregate the market based on ability to pay? Do low-cost plans provide care more efficiently or simply market themselves more effectively to lower-risk subscribers?"

Enthoven's program, they say, is likely to lock the vast majority of patients and physicians into closed panel HMOs run by insurance companies. Finally, they criticize Enthoven's ultimate vision of managed competition - a limited number of huge HMOs managing salaried physicians - as a more radical departure from the current medical-care system than their proposed NHP.

3-C.   Universal Health Care Act of 1991 (HR1300)
(Introduced, March, 1991 by Rep. Marty Russo, D, IL)

To increase access. The federal government (not the states, as would parallel Canada's provincial administration) would administer universal national health insurance for acute and long-term care. However, any state wishing to, could assume administration of its own portion of the plan.

A National Health Trust Fund would receive all funds collected for medical care. Everyone previously under Medicare, Medicaid, CHAMPUS, Veteran's Health Program or any other federal health program would instead be covered by this program. All U.S. citizens would be entitled to identical benefits and free to choose their own doctors, hospital, or medical-care provider. There would be no denial of coverage or penalty because of pre-existing condition or age.

There would be no copayments or deductibles. Providers would be prohibited to charge more than they receive from the government.

Financing. There would be a new 6% payroll tax on employers.

Corporate income taxes would increase from 34% to 38% for businesses with more than $75,000 in profits.

Personal income tax rates would increase from 15%-28%-31% to 15%-30%-34%, with a top rate at 38% for families with incomes over $200,000.

In addition, consumers would pay a premium for long-term care health insurance equal to the present part B premium of Medicare, plus $25 per month for the elderly with incomes above 120% of the poverty level.

Social Security benefits classified as taxable income would rise from 50% to 85%.

States would make payments equal to 85% of their Medicaid cost plus an annual per capita fee of $85.

The federal government would contribute the current amount it spends on medical care.

Cost containment. *Macro-rationing* - The Secretary of HHS would establish, prospectively, annual national and state health budgets. The Secretary would also establish separate budgets for capital expenses and medical education. The national health budget would increase each year, based on inflation and growth of the GNP. A designated government agency would be the "single payer" and would annually negotiate prospective overall budgets with hospitals and nursing homes. Other medical-care facilities, as well as home and community-based services, could elect to be reimbursed by global budgets, fee schedules, or any other prospective payment system, including capitation, provided the designated federal agency approves their choice. Physicians and other medical-care professionals would be reimbursed according to fee schedules established by the HHS Secretary.

Micro-rationing - Research results on outcomes and practice guidelines would be applied to the entire medical-care system.

Administrative savings from uniform claim processing were estimated at $40 billion per year.

Comments. The Russo program would cover basic medical-care services, dental and vision service, prescription drugs, nursing-care facilities, hospice care, and home and community-based services for persons who have difficulty performing at least two activities of daily living.

Proponents say that in 1989 this plan would have reduced total medical-care spending from $589 to $549 billion - a savings of $40 billion. Costs to business would have increased by $23 billion, because of the new payroll tax and the increase in the corporate income tax. Costs for the non-elderly would have decreased by $25 billion, and for the elderly, $33 billion. State and local government would have saved $7 billion; the program would have been cost-neutral to the federal government.

While costs to business would increase initially under the Russo program, elimination of the unbridled escalation of medical-care costs eventually would lower business spending on medical care and remove it as a competitive disadvantage, both internationally and domestically.

Monthly contributions of the elderly living above 120% of the poverty level would increase, as would, in many cases, the taxation of their Social Security benefits. However, in return the elderly would receive long-term care, and elimination of Medicare deductibles and cost-sharing, as well as the need for Medigap insurance.

Senators Wofford (D-PA), Daschle, Wellstone (D- MN), Metzenbaum (D-OH) and Simon (D-IL) introduced a companion Bill to Congressman Russo's Universal Health Care Act of 1991 into the Senate. Congressman Stark introduced a bill for a similar program into the house in 1992. Senator John Kerrey's HealthUSA program, which he supported in his unsuccessful campaign for the 1992 Democratic presidential nomination, was similar to Russo's plan, except it more clearly favored pre-paid managed care such as HMOs over independent, fee-for-service medical practice.

Congressman Russo lost his bid for re-election in 1993, but 70 Congressmen, led by McDermott (D-Wash.) and Conyers (D-Mich.) re-introduced his Universal Health Care Act into the House of Representatives in 1993 as HR 1200.

3-D.   *American Health Security Act*
(A Canadian-like, single-payer proposal, very similar to the Russo Program above, introduced to the Senate in April 1992 (S. 2513) by Sens. Wofford and Daschle and reintroduced in 1993 (S.491) with Sens. Metzenbaum, Wellstone and Simon as cosponsors, and presented in 1993 to the House by 70 Congressmen - see immediately above under comments.)

To increase access. A Federal Health Board (modeled after the Federal Reserve Board) would administer and determine specific services covered by the proposed public program which would be available to everyone.

An independent National Expenditures Board would be established to set a minimum package of covered services including long-term care. This is in contrast to Canada, where administration is by the provinces.

Each state would establish its own public, nonprofit agency to provide comprehensive coverage to everyone. However, if states wished to contract with private insurers to administer their programs, this would be permitted.

Community and migrant health centers and national health service corps would be expanded.

Financing. Individuals and businesses would pay a single premium to the National Expenditure Board, which would distribute the proceeds to the state agencies.

Funds currently provided in the federal budget for Medicare, Medicaid and CHAMPUS would be directed to the National Expenditure Board.

States would help finance their part of the public plan, which would be financed 80% by the federal government, with an amount equivalent to their current contribution to Medicaid, plus an amount to provide their adequate share of support.

Cost containment. *Macro-rationing* - An overall national budget for medical-care spending would be set by the National Expenditures Board. The state agencies would negotiate operating and capital budgets with hospitals and other facilities and fees with doctors.

Micro-rationing - Managed-care plans would be encouraged and outcomes research expanded.

Tort reform would be undertaken.

3-E. "Health Choice" Act (HR 5514) by Reps. John Dingell (D-Mich.) and Henry Waxman (D-Cal.) (Presented to Congress June 30, 1992)

To increase access. A governmental health insurance program would cover everyone and would replace Medicare and Medicaid.

Doctors would be given incentives to practice primary care and in underserved areas.

The National Health Service Corps, and Community and Migrant Health Centers would receive increased funding.

Out-patient prescription drugs would be covered.

Patients could choose plans and providers.

Financing. A 10% value-added-tax (VAT) would be placed on goods and services, excepting food, medical and housing expenses.

Employers would pay a five percent payroll tax.

States would contribute a fixed percentage of their Medicaid costs.

Cost containment. *Macro-rationing* - The government would be the "single payer" that could limit hospital charges and doctors' fees, and reducing administrative complexity. Any rise in health spending would be capped to a level of yearly increase conforming to the rise in GNP. This reform is to be achieved by 1998.

Micro-rationing - Everyone would have to pay deductibles and have copayments for services, but annual out-of-pocket payments would be capped at $2000 per person or $3000 per family. The poor would have their payments subsidized. Individuals would be given incentive to choose a managed-care plan such as HMOs rather than fee-for-service care.

Tort reform would be introduced and alternative systems to resolve malpractice disputes would be tested.

Expand Medicare to Everyone

These programs are similar to the Canadian-style ones comprising category three, except that these programs would expand the Medicare structure to cover the entire population and be the vehicle for federal universal health insurance.

4-A.   The USHealth Act (Presented 1991 by Rep. Roybal for the House Committee on Aging)

To increase access. Medicare would be extended to all Americans regardless of age or income.

Medicare would be expanded to provide long-term care and any other essential medical care service not now covered by Medicare.

Medicare, Medicaid, and private insurance would be consolidated into a single insurance system with Medicare as the foundation. A USHealth Administration would replace the Health Care Financing Administration (HCFA) as the administrative agency.

Financing. Increased revenue will be obtained from the payroll tax by removing the current wage cap. Then the higher earners will pay tax on their entire income.

States would pay half the cost of premiums for their poor. Employers would pay the amount, in the aggregate, of what they now pay to private insurers.

A special surcharge would be placed on all existing corporate and personal income taxes, based on estimates of total national costs of the program and the total of revenues to be received from a) and b) above.

Cost containment. *Macro-rationing* - USHealth would put a cap on the nation's medical-care costs equal to 13% of GNP. Within that 13%, the program would set a sub-cap for long-term care of 1.1% of GNP. Providers would be paid prospectively, using the Medicare DRG and RBRVS mechanisms indexed to the growth in GNP.

Micro-rationing - Beneficiaries would pay co-insurance of 20% for medical and skilled nursing care, and 25% for non-skilled long-term care. These copayments would be limit ed to $600 per person annually for short term, catastrophic illnesses and to $1000 per person per year for long term illnesses. Both the poor and those who choose managed-care plans would be exempt from cost-sharing.

The Medicare model to cover everyone would save $30 billion per year. That would be so because Medicare currently returns significantly more in benefits per dollar invested than private programs.

Comment. The House Committee on Aging considered the Pepper Commission proposal a plausible alternative to their USHealth plan.

4-B.   Mediplan Health Care Act of 1991 (HR650) (introduced by Representative Pete Stark [D-Cal] in Jan. 1991)

To increase access. National health insurance, by expanding Medicare to include all residents of the United States, whether citizens or not, would give universal access. The name Medicare would be changed to "Mediplan".

The benefits for everyone would be the same as currently under Part A and Part B of Medicare, as well as special preventive care for children and pregnant women. There would be no deductibles or copayments.

Previously contracted private health plans would continue. They would be required to provide any contracted health benefits that were above Mediplan benefits.

Financing. Everyone except those currently Medicare-eligible would pay a basic income tax for Mediplan, in addition to any payroll tax paid by employers. The basic income tax for Mediplan would be either $1000 ($2000 for joint returns) or 12.5% of gross income over $8000 ($16000 for joint returns) whichever is less. There would be an additional tax of 2% of any gross income over $16000 ($32000 for joint returns).

Corporate tax-payers and tax-exempt organizations would pay two percent of gross income to Mediplan.

Employers would pay a payroll tax of 40 cents an hour for hourly employees, and 10% of salaried employees, up to $800 per employee per year.

States would be required to maintain their present Medicaid payments for Mediplan, increased yearly in line with the consumer price index (CPI).

Cost containment. *Macro-rationing* - Mediplan would include application of current Medicare payment rules, including DRGs and RBRVSs.

Micro-rationing - There would be a single annual deductible of $500, and the same copayments as currently under Medicare. The limit on out-of-pocket expenses, including deductibles, co-insurance and copayments would be $2500 per year. Those with incomes under 100% of the poverty level would be exempt from all such payments, and those under 200% of the poverty level would have their cost-sharing indexed accordingly.

In April 1992, Congressman Stark submitted an additional proposal for streamlining administrative expenses. HR 4956 provides that the Department of HHS set up a national system of electronic health cards and regional clearing houses to take over the work done by individual insurers.

Comment. Mediplan makes no provisions for long-term care.

4-C.   Health Care America (the AARP Proposal)

To increase access. Health Care America would expand Medicare to cover everyone, regardless of job status. It would encompass the full spectrum medical-care benefits, including prescription drugs, dental and long-term care, and preventive medicine programs, especially for children.

Medicaid would be abolished.

No one would be excluded because of pre-existing conditions.

Patients would be free to choose their care-providers.

Financing. Everyone who could afford it would contribute $50 per month.

Employers would either pay an 8% payroll tax or provide employees and dependents with equivalent or better coverage.

Employees in such a private plan would pay no more than 20% of the premium.

$112 billion estimated to be needed for 1993 would be obtained from added revenues. These revenues would come from a 100% increase in sin taxes on alcohol and tobacco, a 5% surtax on corporate incomes and an increased tax on large estates. A special tax of 3% on incomes over $15,000 for the individual and $20,000 for families, or a new 5% value-added tax for goods and services could provide the rest of any needed funds. The VAT would not be for food, medical services or housing, and would be refunded for low-income persons.

Cost containment. *Macro-rationing* - Health Care America would set national and state spending budgets, as well as standard rates for acute and long-term providers. It would also place strict limits on prescription drug prices.

Micro-rationing - Deductible for acute hospital care would be $200 per individual and $400 per family. There would be a 10% co-insurance premium for out-patient physician, surgical and mental health services, laboratory services and prescription drugs. Individuals would pay $600 per year for Medicare coverage. Long-term care would require a 20% co-insurance for home and community-based services and a 35% co-insurance for nursing home care. However, total individual cost would be capped at $1500 annually and family costs at $3000. Low-income persons would not have to pay any copayments or deductibles.

Comment. Some AARP council members did not believe the country was ready for a single payer, national health insurance system, even though they thought it would be the simplest and eventually least costly program, even if it required greater funding, and more taxation, "up front". However, after a year's discussion with the membership and in deference to the many who favored a single-payer system, the AARP legislative council decided to present their program in two forms: a "blended plan" as detailed above, and a single-payer one, in which everyone is covered under one publicly financed insurance program. Under the single-payer plan the government would serve as the sole insurer for health services.

Most observers, even the AMA and several legislators who had their own programs, were favorable to the AARP proposal. The American Hospital Association was critical, be cause the cost control features of the AARP program "would put the hospitals in a financial bind and impair quality care."

(It should be noted that, in the following tables, constructed to outline the data in this chapter, it is impossible to include all the variations in each category of proposed programs and remain succinct. Nevertheless, the tables do present the major items of each, and can serve as a concise summary for ready comparison between them.)

Table V-1
Market Reform Programs
(Tax Credits to Buy Private Insurance)

1. Access:

    a. Middle class - tax-credits for health insurance premiums
    b. self-employed: 100% tax deduction for health insurance
    c. poor and near-poor: vouchers to buy health insurance
    d. reform insurance industry: community-rated premiums for small firms; no exclusion for previous health

2. Cost containment:

    a. Medicaid payments for acute care to be capped
    b. managed care incentive (through medical-care accounts)
    c. tort reform
    d. administrative reform

3. Financing:

    extra $28 to 40 billion required annually in taxes

Table V-2
Market Reform Programs
(Republican Party Proposal)

In Favor:

1. augment rather than replaces current system (preserves insurance industry)
2. access expanded:

   a) to all uninsured
   b) reforms insurance industry to eliminate exclusions and experience rating

3. lowers costs:

   a) tort and administrative reforms
   b) favoring of managed care
   c) capping Medicaid payments

Against:

1. universal access unlikely
2. adequate insurance still beyond means of poorer 50% of uninsured
3. Do not cover long-term care
4. cost containment unlikely (while favoring competition, incentives for it weak)
5. do not address escalation of costs due to aging and new technology
6. do consumers have enough "know-how" to shop for plans? (people to shop "on own" in private market)
7. Repub. Party does not state how extra costs will be financed ($35 to 40 billion per year)

Table V-3
Mandated Employer Insurance Programs
(Pay-or-Play)

1. Access:

   a. large employers required to buy private insurance for employees or enroll them in public plan and pay tax
   b. small employers to insure employees by public agency (thus get community-rated premiums)
   c. self-employed, retirees under 65 and others not employed to be covered by public agency and pay tax for this
   d. poor and near-poor covered by public agency with government subsidizing premiums

2. Cost containment:

   a. managed competition - knowledgeable firms or government agency to contract with competing plans
   b. managed care - nature of system and government regulation will favor such plans
   c. global budgeting and negotiation with providers endorsed by latest proposals
   d. administrative and tort reform

3. Financing:

   requires an extra $12 to 66 billion annually in taxes.

Table V-4
Employer Insurance Programs
(Democratic Party Proposals)

In Favor:

1. build on present system through which most people get medical care (insurance industry essentially unchanged)

2. access expanded to most uninsured

3. cost containment (better than market reform plans):

   a) managed competition and managed care
   b) global budgeting and single-payer system
   c) administrative and tort reforms

Against:

1. will increase costs to employers and their products
2. public program apt to be less generous than others, leading to "two-tiered care"
3. unemployment could increase
4. achievement of universal access questionable
5. no provision for long-term care
6. cost containment not certain
7. no control of escalation of costs due to aging and new technology
8. requires an extra $12 to 66 billion annually in taxes.

Table V-5
Universal Health Insurance + Managed Competition + Managed Care (Enthoven)

1. To increase access:

   A. large employers to pay 80% of premiums of full-time workers; and to pay 8% of part-timers' wages to public sponsor
   B. small employers pay 8% of payroll to public sponsor
   C. public sponsors - to pay 80% of premiums for those not insured by large employers & enrollee pays 20% + 8% of income; pay up to 100% of premium for poor

2. Financing public sponsor:

   A. 8% payroll tax paid for part-time workers
   B. 8% income tax on individuals not covered by employer
   C. Increased tax revenues from limiting employer deduction to 80% of premiums costs and none by employees

3. Cost containment:

   A. managed competition - large employers and public sponsors contract with competing "qualified" health plans
   B. managed-care plans to be favored by tax policy

4. Comments:

   A. expands access (but not likely to be universal unless an increase in taxes - $80 billion)
   B. feasibility good since present insurance system is preserved
   C. proposers claim increased competition will keep it budget neutral and save too
   D. will add to business costs and products
   E. long-term care not covered
   F. No way for controlling acceleration of costs due to aging and innovations

Table V-6
Universal National Health Insurance Programs

1. Access:

   a) universal
   b) long-term care included
   c) no copayments or deductibles, nor denial of coverage for any reason

2. Cost containment:

   a) single-payer system
   b) global prospective budgeting
   c) reduced administrative expense

3. Financing:

   by taxation on business and individuals (as in Canada)

Table V-7
Universal National Health Insurance Programs

In Favor:

1. universal access guaranteed
2. cost containment more certain than relying on increased competition
3. acceleration of costs due to age and technology controlled
4. administrative complexity reduced
5. stress on business reduced: cost of products and labor negotiations
6. free choice of doctor
7. private practice preserved instead of managed care
8. more affluent pay proportionately more than do less affluent for same care

Against:

1. increases government bureaucracy
2. the possibility that government will dictate treatment decisions
3. the possibility of need for the queue to control access to non-emergency high-tech services
4. not politically feasible for United States (too big a change; $250 billion in extra taxes, even if recovered from private)

Chapter VI

The Political Realities of Health-care Reform

What is the political feasibility of the various programs for solving the U.S. medical-care crisis?

Any answer to this question must consider the potency of entrenched interests in the medical-care industry and the extent of change these interests will tolerate. The medical-care industry is the largest in the United States. Accounting for one-seventh of the national economy, it employs more people than any other sector of the economy: ten million by 1992, an increase of 43% in 4 years. Also, it is the projected largest source of new jobs through the next decade. The health insurance industry alone takes in annually $280 billion in premiums, and employs about 460,000 people. It has grown in recent years particularly because of the enlargement of health delivery organizations, such as HMOs, it owns and operates.

The medical-care industry also includes a number of entrepreneurial firms who own and operate large hospital chains and entities for the delivery of diagnostic and therapeutic medical care. Hospital employees and hospital associations have strong lobbying arms. Physicians too have an entrenched financial interest in the current medical-care delivery system, and well-financed organizations to represent them. Of course, the pharmaceutical industry as well has mushroomed, and will likely continue to do so.

While all medical-care workers have a vested interest in the *status quo*, several physicians' organizations - including the prestigious

117

American College of Physicians - publicly supported radical reform of the U.S. health system, favoring universal national health insurance and a single-payer system (see Chapter V). No one questions that the proposed medical-care reforms will cost jobs, particularly in small businesses. The most likely to be adopted programs will oblige many companies to offer health cover age for the first time, undoubtedly forcing some of them to fold.

In addition to those economically affected, there are many people who, despite dismay at the size of their present medical bills, would oppose any changes depriving them of the prompt and truly superb care they now receive. This well-insured portion of society includes increasing numbers of the elderly who are accustomed to the abundance of expensive care provided by Medicare and supplemented by Medigap insurance, which is affordable to many of the aged. Those opposed to radical reform of the current U.S. medical-care system have large sums available for lobbying which assure them a careful hearing by legislators, who need to raise at least $2000 a week while in office to finance re-election campaigns.

In 1989, when the 15 member Pepper Commission reported back to Congress with its recommendation to alter the medical-care delivery system, it was declared "dead on arrival". This was because the Commission's congressional members did not think their constituents realized the gravity of the nation's medical-care crisis. Most Americans, being well-insured, believed the crisis was some body else's business and there was no point for Congress to take a stand on a reform which would only bring them more taxes.

One and a half years later the situation was markedly different. Polls indicated the concern over medical care had risen in the public consciousness. Not only were increasingly large numbers of uninsured people, but the middle class were finding that their insurance did not protect them against the rising costs of medical care, or that their employers and insurers were cutting back on their benefits. Many people working for small businesses or with pre-existing conditions were finding health insurance prohibitively expensive, or unavailable.

Thus while the medical-care crisis still ranked below issues of national security and the economy, it was now on a par with education, poverty and the homeless. Pennsylvanian Harris Wofford's unexpected victory after a 1991 senatorial campaign based on his promises of medical-care reform showed the 1992 congressional and presidential candidates how greatly the medical-care crisis loomed in the public mind.

In addition, the detrimental effect of medical-care costs on the economy was causing large businesses to support government intervention. Large corporations complained that their workers' health insurance had become a major factor in their products' costs, hindering their competitive position in the international marketplace. The large manufacturers consequently became a potent countervailing force to the insurance companies in the struggle over solutions to the crisis in medical care.

But despite the widespread agreement on the need to reform, there was no consensus on how to finance any of the solutions. How large a tax increase - even if it were a transfer from out-of-pocket spending - would the public support? The least radical reforms - based on market reforms or a play-or-pay managed-competition program - would need $50 to 70 billion in up front money to pay for universal access. That sum would not even cover oft-mentioned items like drugs, or long term or psychiatric care. The American electorate has repeatedly demonstrated its antipathy to tax increases, but the already enormous national debt inhibits any further borrowing to finance medical-care reform.

Rationing presents another important obstacle to medical-care reform. Rationing is the only way to control the escalation in costs caused by the increase in necessary care generated by the aging of the population and introduction of new technology. But since the term "rationing" has a pejorative connotation, including any such proposal adversely affects the chances for acceptance of any reform program. However, if politicians and planners made the distinction between unnecessary and necessary care when considering cost containment, they might be able to regulate unnecessary care, even though they wouldn't be able to ration necessary care.

On the other hand, a society could decide that it preferred to apportion its wealth to unlimited medical care instead of spending it on multiple cars, homes, and bathrooms, plus the myriad of other consumer products available to an affluent nation. That would make medical-care rationing unnecessary, but such an hypothesis is pure fantasy.

Both major political parties endorsed managed competition and managed care as well as tort and administrative reforms in the 1992 presidential campaign. Somewhat belatedly, the Democratic Party mentioned global budgeting, evoking criticism from the Republicans that such budgeting would lead to rationing. The Republican criticism is almost certainly true, since effective global budgeting will entail not only elimination of unnecessary care and administrative and malpractice costs be reduced, but also, for long-term effectiveness, some rationing of necessary care.

Global budgeting - the imposition of caps - also is problematic because it would apply only to programs paid for by government, which account for only 43% of total health expenditures (29% on Medicare and Medicaid plus 14% on other programs). That leaves 57% of expenditures in the private sector untouched. Also, legislation to cap private sector spending could be challenged on constitutional grounds.

In addition, legislators considering reforming the medical- care system know that any cuts, even just to make it more efficient, will jostle employment, companies, and even whole industries. Such dislocations would place added strain on an economy already reeling from scaling back the defense industry after the demise of the Cold War. The vociferous constituent complaints about closing unnecessary military bases surely give them a taste of just how strong a reaction the dislocations caused by medical-care reform would summon forth.

Anyone wishing to reform the medical-care system must consider how much shift in basic political ideology our nation will tolerate. The least radical change from our present system - to a state controlled social insurance system like those in France, Germany or the Netherlands - is not at all feasible. While those systems afford universal access and cost less than our system, they all evolved slowly over the past century from voluntary social welfare societies and would be impossible to replicate quickly. These systems demand two things - a good supply of general practitioners, and strong doctor-patient relationships - in order to effect implicit rationing. Both are in short supply in the United States.

Perhaps the American public can tolerate only incremental changes evolving slowly toward universal coverage and better cost containment, but not a sudden overhaul of the entire system. Reports of queuing in Canada and especially in Great Britain add to the ranks of opponents of any complete nationalization of medical care here. Indeed, even many pragmatists abroad believe any national system must provide an "escape hatch" to private care for the minority - 10% in the U.K. - that are affluent and vocal, lest they spread discontent with any system denying them something, no matter how effective that system overall. But any such reform that might openly accede to such tiering here would evoke strong protest from egalitarians so outspoken in the United States, even though that bit of tiering would replace the greater injustices caused by the present marketplace rationing. Furthermore, practitioners and planners will always disagree about treatment that's not cost-effective epidemiologically and yet helps specific individuals. The "rule-of-rescuc" operates almost everywhere, and particularly among the more affluent and aware.

Despite the reports of queuing in Canada, many programs proposed for the United States would emulate the Canadian national health insurance system. Its proponents claim the greater resources already devoted to medical care in the United States would preclude queuing here. These proponents intend not to lower the percentage of GDP that goes to medical care, but to prevent its escalation beyond the 13.2% of GDP expended in 1991. By 1993, several bills had been introduced into Congress similar to the Canadian system but neither of the political parties supported so radical an alteration of the U.S. delivery system.

There are a number of other reasons why nationalization of health insurance in United States does not seem feasible. Nationalization would nearly eliminate the private health insurance industry. Doctors, hospitals, unions and suppliers would oppose and lobby against such a change. Taxes necessary for nationalization - an estimated $250 to $400 billion - would not be politically feasible, even though they would actually constitute a transfer from the less visible spending in the private sector. Others say the Canadian system is too egalitarian for the United States, that the affluent, not wanting to be treated the same as the poor, would militate against the change. Finally, social development in the United States means that large, well-insured segments of the population - especially the politically- potent elderly, are used to abundant, prompt care. No universally-available system can supply that kind of care, and still permanently contain costs. It is services to the aged, in particular, that are subjected to implicit micro-rationing in national health systems abroad.

The fact that the two major problems in the U.S. medical-care crisis conflict makes its solution much more difficult. Solving the first problem, achieving universal access, aggravates the second difficulty, the system's escalating costs. Moreover, the cost of medical care continues to be a major contributor to the overwhelming economic problem in the United States, our enormous national debt. But to accomplish any health system reform, the government would have to invest many billions up front, especially for insuring the uninsured. To raise this money, the government would have to either impose large taxes or increase the national debt. But interest payment on the debt in 1992 had already reached $293 billion, and was seriously harming the national economy.

Reducing the national debt and coping with medical-care costs can be accomplished only by raising taxes and/or curtailing expenditures. In the 1992 presidential election both parties tacitly acknowledged that neither alternative constituted a viable political platform. And neither Republicans nor Democrats went beyond generalities in their programs for medical-care reform or for reducing the governmental debt. As though by mutual consent, they did not prod each other too greatly on the details for combating these problems. Thus the existence of the massive national debt has been a principal barrier to meaningful health reform.

The Republican approach, as promulgated by then-President Bush during his campaign for re-election, would be least disturbing to the existing medical-care delivery system. Instead of meeting the crisis in medical care by increased governmental regulation, the Republican approach would enhance market forces, using incentives to increase access to medical care. Moderate and low-income people would receive tax-credits - permission to deduct premiums from their income taxes - for buying health insurance. The poor would receive vouchers to buy insurance. The Republicans would enact rules for private insurers to stabilize coverage for those already insured. Such proposals would cover at least half of those uninsured, but many analysts said the tax credit for people with incomes up to 150% of the poverty level was inadequate, and millions would still be unable to buy insurance. While the Republican programs promote managed care and administrative and malpractice reforms that could lower medical-care costs, they have no proposals to control the more important causes of the unbridled escalation in the cost of medical care: inordinate charges by providers, insurer profits, and the constant increase in necessary care due to the aging of the population and the development of technological innovations.

The play-or-pay programs put forward by the Democratic Party proposed to move toward universal access by offering a public agency to supplement private insurers. Coverage by the public agency for those not insured by their employer would be very attractive, but not mandatory. The public agency would consist either of an expanded Medicare program, an entirely new agency, or possibly one created simply to oversee health insurance industry reform. In any case, the Democrats would regulate the insurance industry to provide continuity and guaranteed renewability of coverage,as well as community rating of premiums instead of experience. The private health insurance industry would be pre served.

In addition, the Democratic program included several cost control measures including: managed-care plans, coordination and simplification of administrative procedures, reduction of drug costs, prevention of unnecessary duplication of high technology equipment, and reform of liability disputes. In an attempt to control the escalation in costs, some Democratic Party programs in the fall of 1992 proposed managed competition and a National Board (consisting of providers, payers and consumers) to set global budget targets for, and oversee, negotiations between providers and purchasers. However, no program mentioned that global budgeting would eventually necessitate micro-rationing. Nor was it mentioned that the United States lacked the infrastructure used abroad for this purpose - the corps of general practitioners, and the well-established doctor-patient relationships.

During the 1992 presidential campaign, both parties gave more details on their approach to increasing access to medical care than on their ideas for cost-containment. Democratic programs did address the cost-containment problem more actively than did the Republicans. But neither party mentioned that any program would initially require increased taxes, no matter how great the eventual savings. The Republican tax-credit and voucher proposal was estimated to require $35 to $40 billion annually in new taxes - about the same amount required by the least-expensive Democratic play-or-pay or managed-competition program. Replacing private insurance premiums with a government administered national insurance program could require as much as $300 to $400 billion of new taxes, though the net medical-care costs would decrease after the transfer of the less visible private sector and individual expenditures to the government.

At the same time, observers commented that the increasing concern of the electorate for cost-containment might make radical changes - even institution of a Canadian-style national health insurance program - more feasible. They cited the Wofford's victory over former Governor Richard Thornburgh in the 1991 Pennsylvania Senatorial race, largely due to Wofford's support of national health insurance. However, Wofford did not provide any details in his campaign. Later, in his senate bill he agreed to permit states to contract with private insurers to administer programs.

In his unsuccessful campaign for the 1992 Democratic presidential nomination, Senator John Kerrey made a proposal for medical-care reform which was even more radical than the Canadian system. He proposed replacing the private practice of medicine with managed care. In support of this proposal, Kerrey stated that HMOs already covered 36.5 million people, or 14.6% of the U.S. population, and that HMOs and PPOs together in 1990 covered 38% of the employed, up from 29% in 1988. Kerrey's proposal, which he called Health USA, did not exclude private health plans, which would have reassured those fearing they would have no choice beyond a large government plan. Kerrey also proposed to reassure HMOs and other such insurers by the large role reserved for them in organizing care, as opposed to the Canadian-style programs that tended to shut them out by preserving private practice.

In summary, entrenched interests and public prejudices against taxes and rationing combined in 1992 to prevent either political party from adopting a program that offered any reform that had proven successful elsewhere. Neither party seriously considered programs which, like those in England and Canada, guaranteed universal access and limited private insurers to a marginal role. Proven cost-containment measures, such as global budgeting and single-payer methods, were mentioned only belatedly by the Democrats and then were attacked by the Republicans for leading to rationing. It is indeed ironic, that in the United States, the bastion of free enterprise, the private practice of medicine is under unprecedented attack, while everywhere abroad - even in the more socially oriented countries of Britain and Scandinavia - it is being vigorously preserved.

Indeed, Czechoslovakian President Vaclav Havel commented in a June 25, 1992 article in the New York Review of Books that what his people need after 40 years of detached attentions in the polyclinics, is the personal attentions of one's own chosen, privately-practicing physician - who should be paid by a new system of general health insurance. The most important aspect of medical care, wrote Havel, is the personal relationship between doctor and patient, and that now is being restored in Czechoslovakia. Ironically, the escalating cost of medical care in the United States is creating a strange ideological alignment that is further eroding the doctor-patient relationship. Private insurance companies and businesses, despite their commitment to free-enterprise and their opposition to government regulation, have used their power over reimbursement to align themselves with government agencies to intrude into individual patient's care and to make decisions about what treatment is appropriate.

While doctors complain bitterly about such third-party intrusion, performed all too often by clerks and nurses, they have nevertheless failed to endorse a Canadian or English-style program, which would limit their incomes but preserve their autonomy. Physicians apparently want both incomes, and their autonomy too; but since their incomes are steadily eroding, perhaps they will change their minds. Indeed, one prestigious organization, The American College of Physicians, has already indicated its support for Canadian-style reform.

By the end of the 1992 presidential campaign, both political parties had converged on a program essentially as proposed by Enthoven: to increase access by an approach combining mandated-employer insurance with government-provided coverage. Cost-containment would rest on Enthoven's managed-competition formulation, and increasing use of the man aged-care concept. These ideas were the least disturbing to the current medical-care financing structure through insurance companies, and closest to the already evolving delivery system through managed-care plans like HMOs. The increased business that would be generated by insuring the nation's 37,000,000 uninsured, either by broader employer coverage or payment by a government agency, made Enthoven's program palatable to the insurance companies. The largest insurance companies already owned HMOs and were using other managed care techniques as well. They saw that the Clinton administration's reforms would only increase that business. In December 1992, the insurance industry officially climbed aboard the managed-care bandwagon when its Health Insurance Association of America (HIA) called for a federal law that would require insurance coverage for all Americans, either through their employers or through the government. The HIA agreed cost-containment should be carried out by a law limiting the tax-deductibility to the cost of a basic policy bought by employers for their employees, or by employees them selves. Such a measure, said the association, would make individuals shop for coverage more carefully, thus increasing competition among insurance companies to attract subscribers by offering the most coverage at the lowest possible rates.

President Clinton after his election made medical-care reform one of his first priorities. He indicated that he would propose to Congress a program based on Enthoven's proposal for universal coverage and cost containment through managed competition, strengthened by global budgets enforced by a National Health Board. That board would both set per capita budgets for states, limiting their public sponsors' expenditures, and set caps on health insurance premiums for all sponsors, public or private. Where competition among plans was not possible, as for example in sparsely populated rural areas, states would regulate providers' fees in order to meet their budgets.

The Clinton administration was also considering proposing price controls on drugs, doctors and hospitals, requirements on the health insurance industry to offer community rating of premiums, tort reform, and taxing medical-care plans offering more than basic benefits. Proceeds from these taxes would be used to cover many uninsured employees, through tax credits to small businesses to offset their proposed payroll tax for health insurance. Control of drug prices would be popular, because they are paid for mostly "out-of-pocket". But since drugs account for only 8% of medical-care costs, the greatest debate appeared likely to center on how else to finance the administration's reform proposal, whose initial cost for universal access would be an estimated $70 and 82 billion a year. The final cost would depend on what benefits would be included in addition to those for basic acute care. For example, long-term care for only home assistance would add $8-15 billion, mental health and addictive care $4-7 billion, prescription drugs $8-10 billion, and for prevention and treatment of common dental diseases in children and adults, $7.1 billion.

By 1993, the Clinton administration was considering a variety of taxes to finance medical-care reform. An increase in sin taxes, for example, would yield only about $10 billion a year, but a VAT of 5% should yield $50 billion. Taxing health plans that provide benefits beyond the basic might generate $25 billion annually. A five percent surcharge on all income taxes would raise $26 billion a year; a three percent surtax on hospitals and doctors would yield $10 billion annually. Finally, raising the taxation on Social Security benefits from 50% to 85% for single recipients with incomes over $25000 and $32000 for couples would generate $1.7 billion in 1994 and cost each such recipient $500.

However, many of these taxes were already earmarked for budget deficit reduction, as was a $69 billion reduction in Medicare expenditures over five years originally proposed to finance medical-care reform. The proposed reductions in Medicare would mostly be borne by providers, but also would include reduction in the yearly cost-of-living increases (COLA). Furthermore, the prospect of a payroll tax of 7 or 8%, as suggested in Enthoven's play-or-pay, managed-competition, managed-care proposal, frightened small businesses.

Thus, radical reforms will become feasible only if the program of managed competition - which has no previous track record any where - fails to contain escalation in costs or to provide adequate and satisfying care. Such radical reforms would mean turning to nationalized systems already proven effective abroad in both providing adequate medical care to an entire population and still containing expenditures better than the United States. However, yet another circumstance could forestall such an eventuality: proponents of managed competition have made it clear that it would take a decade to attain its objectives. Thus, even if managed competition does not work in its first few years, its proponents will likely demand it continue.

But even if it should become apparent that managed competition is not the answer to the medical-care crisis, it still would take a long time to successfully emulate systems abroad. That is because these systems depend upon large numbers of general practitioners and good doctor-patient relationships. Recapturing those pre-conditions here is bound to be a slow process.

Today, the discouragement with previous gradual changes and widespread opinion that change is urgently needed combine to make radical reform seem the only practical option for correcting the U.S. medical care system. But - despite everyone's impatience - continuing steady incremental changes rather than immediate total reform might well be the way to achieve a system that will best satisfy the American people. Further efforts, i.e., to eliminate provider and patient incentives to overutilize resources; to reduce administrative and other operational expenditures; to make primary care more attractive to physicians, could well produce a satisfactory system that could also afford universal care. And such an incremental approach could well be more acceptable than taxing the public to provide for an immediate, revolutionary reform.

Table VI-1
Items Bearing on Political Feasibility
of Health Care Reform

Working Against Reform:

1. potency of entrenched interests: insurers, providers, drug industry
2. economic effect of cutting back an industry
3. increasing access entails greater costs
4. any reform requires increased taxation
5. permanent cost containment requires some form of new rationing
6. reforms increase governmental regulation
7. options for change require evolving renewed or new infrastructure

In favor of reform:

1. numbers of people without access increasing
2. benefits being cut for those insured
3. health costs can diminish business competitiveness
4. contribution of health costs to national debt

Table VI-2
Anomalies in Discussion of Health Care Reform

1. Presidential candidates did not vie over details of reform
2. Taxes unacceptable for health care reform even if, eventually, a saving for all
3. Rationing never mentioned by proposers of programs for health care reform, but every nation does it
4. Private practice preserved in more welfare oriented nations abroad but its demise agreed upon in United States

GLOSSARY

Accountable Health Partnerships (or plans): synonym for qualified health plans; used by Jackson Hole Group. Actually, what they envision are vertical networks, comprehending primary through tertiary hospital care, competing for contracts with "sponsors".

Adverse selection: the situation in which the sickest members of society can only purchase very expensive insurance (expensive because they are at high risk of using it), while the healthy (often young) remain uncovered or enroll in less costly plans and use less care (see "community, or social insurance, rates" and "casualty rates").

Ambulatory care: see primary care.

Appropriateness of service studies: see "outcomes research".

Asset protection program: permits individuals who purchase long-term care insurance (which would be tax-deductible to them) to be able to protect designated assets, up to the dollar value of their insurance benefits, from being included in any eligibility determination for Medicaid coverage for long-term care.

Basic medical care (or basic benefits): (specified by the federal HMO Act) includes physician services, inpatient and outpatient hospital services, emergency health services, x-rays and laboratory services, mental health services (limited), treatment for drug and alcohol abuse, home health services and certain preventive health services. Most other concepts of "basic benefits" do not include psychiatric treatment or substance abuse programs. Inherent in all perceptions of basic care is that treatments without proven effectiveness ("outcome") are not included. Also, treatments not necessary for essential health, such as cosmetic surgery, are not included.

Capitation: a method of payment (used by HMOs), in which patients (or their insurers) pay a flat annual fee, per person, to a provider of services regardless of how many services any one patient consumes;

the object is to shift the economic risk in controlling resource utilization to the provider.

Case-managed care: see "primary care network".

Casualty rated insurance (experience-rated, individually rated, risk-rated, actuarial-rated or conventional insurance): casualty insurance with casualty-rated premiums, when applied to health insurance, is usually called insurance with experience-rated premiums or experience-rated insurance. It sets premiums according to the expected cost of claims by individual applicants, based on the likelihood of their need for medical care in the reasonably foreseeable future. Thus rates can be kept down by the exclusion of individuals based on their previous health status, age, sex, occupation and/or geographic location, or charging them much higher, and generally non-affordable rates if their risk is in creased by one of the afore-mentioned factors. Also, small groups - such as employees of small businesses - would be charged higher rates than very large groups, such as represented by employees of large corporations, because the possibility of a small number of high-risk individuals in a small group could be costly to the insurer as opposed to their being submerged in the greater numbers of a large organization.

Catastrophic health insurance: a separate insurance policy, or an added feature of some policies, that protects against the cost of illness that would exceed the limits of an ordinary policy; not to be confused with long-term care.

Certificate-of-need program (CON): This program demands that sizable capital expenditures be approved by a governmental agency and a certificate-of-need be issued before a hospital can make an addition or alteration, or acquire expensive new equipment.

Cherry-picking: a term applied to the procedure of insurers and managed-care organizations seeking out only individuals who are healthy risks to enter into their plan (refusing to cover those who are not).

133

Cognitive activity: activity of physicians based on their knowledge or thinking; as opposed to doing, such as a "procedure".

Co-insurance: share of premium paid by employee in an employer sponsored insurance program.

Community-rated Insurance (also known as assessment insurance): as opposed to experience-rated or casualty insurance premiums, community-rated insurance premiums are uniform for all - regardless of individual or group risks - and thus the rate is set by the exposure to risk of the entire population - the young and healthy having higher rates (than would be their casualty-rated premium) supporting the unhealthy and old whose rates are lowered from what they would be, if casualty-rated.

Competitive Medical Organizations (CMOs): are outgrowths of successful HMOs. They are voluntary, vertically integrated, regionally based, non-profit or for-profit, managed-care health delivery systems in which providers collaborate to provide comprehensive medical services. The key component is a primary care focused, but multi-specialty, group which might contract with affiliated independent physicians. Secondary care is through community hospitals with high technology services being provided by smaller, regional tertiary hospitals. An example is the Kaiser Foundation in California.

Conditional coverage: a recent concept of the health insurance industry in an effort to control the costs of paying for the use of new technologies. It proposes to pay for limited use of a new technology only in settings like selected medical centers where data on its effectiveness can be generated.

Consumers: in terms of medical-care, consumers are patients, or organizations: such as employers or insurance companies, when acting to purchase services (from providers or plans offering provider services) to be supplied to patients.

Continuity-of-care: means that a patient is repeatedly cared for by the same doctor.

Coordinated care: term used by the Bush administration for managed care.

Co-payment: requirement that an insured individual pay a fixed percentage of the costs of services provided; usually 20% under Medicare.

Cost-effectiveness studies: an epidemiological term; relates effectiveness of a treatment for patients in relationship to its financial cost to the community or nation.

Cost outliers: In prospective payment to hospitals for individual care (as in DRGs) this term identifies those patients whose costs for care far exceeds the average for their diagnosis.

Cost-shifting: Term used to describe the activity of providers when they spread (or add) the costs of a service or services given non-paying, uninsured patients to those of their paying patients (usually insured).

Day-outliers: In prospective payment to hospitals for individual care (as in DRGs) this term identifies those patients whose length of stay far exceeds the average for their diagnosis.

Deductible: a set amount of medical expenses a patient must pay before becoming eligible for insurance benefits.

Defensive medicine: ordering diagnostic tests or doing procedures in the practice of medicine not indicated for the health or welfare of the patient, but rather ordered, or done, by the practitioner as self-protection in anticipation of a possible malpractice suit, should the patient ever initiate one.

Diagnostic related groups (DRGs) system: In the DRG system all patients insured by Medicare are classified into one of 467 groups according to: diagnosis on admission to the hospital, age and sex, whether the treatment is medical or surgical, and whether there are secondary diagnoses. Hospitals are then reimbursed, prospectively, on the basis of the patient's diagnosis; if the hospital expends more than the DRG allows, it must absorb the loss; conversely, it may keep any overage from the DRG payment above its actual cost. It is a method that provides incentive to hospitals to be more cost- conscious in the care of patients, including discharging them as soon as possible.

DRG creep: diagnoses of hospitalized patients placed in categories better remunerated than the ones that better fits their conditions.

Employee Retirement and Income Security Act (ERISA): passed in 1974, reserves to the federal authority sole power to regulate the field of employee benefit plans. It does not preempt states' right to regulate insurance.

Enterprise liability: a tort reform plan that shifts responsibility for negligence from individual physicians to the enterprises through which they give care, such as an HMO.

Experience-rated insurance: see casualty rated insurance.

Explicit rationing: is when specific items of medical care, and for whom, are prescribed by law or public edict and therefore is "visible" to all.

Fee schedule creep: giving a service to a patient, or describing it, in a category better remunerated than in one that would be more appropriate under the circumstance - as doing, or reporting, an "extended office visit" instead of a "routine office visit".

Freedom-of-choice: a principle which states that patients (consumers) should be permitted to choose their own physicians or facilities for care (providers).

Fund holder: name for those general practitioners in the British NHS who are budgeted a total of funds yearly and which is to be administered by them to pay for all the medical care of patients on their lists; to be fund holders, practitioners (usually a group) must have a patient list of at least 9000 (as originally planned); any funds left over at the end of a year can be used to add to, or improve, the services their practices can offer their patients; over-spending in any one year has to be made up by the next year's budget.

Gap insurance: insurance policy to reimburse holder for copayments and/or deductibles demanded by primary health insurer or for services not covered by primary insurer; also called secondary or supplementary insurance, or for persons covered by Medicare often called "65 special" or medigap insurance.

Global budgeting: is when the total amounts expended on medical care (or an item of care) is prospectively restricted; often through a single-payer mechanism for negotiation with providers - usually by, or with the participation, of government; often referred to as "expenditure caps" (not to be confused with price & wage controls).

Gross domestic product (GDP): the total monetary value of all goods produced and services provided in a country during one year.

Gross national product (GNP): is the gross domestic product plus receipts by U.S. residents of interest and dividends and reinvest ed earnings of foreign affiliates of U.S. corporations less payments to foreign residents of interest and dividends and reinvest ed earnings of U.S. affiliates of foreign corporations.

Health care: refers to preventive care as well as medical care (q.v.); also concerned with social and economic factors impinging on the health of people.

Health Care Financing Agency (HCFA): the part of HHS that administers and regulates Medicare and Medicaid.

Health Insurance Purchasing Cooperative (HIPC): same as "public sponsor" of Enthoven program (Chapter V-2A); also called "Purchasing Alliance".

Health Maintenance Organization (HMO): enroll subscribers who pay a single fee as insurance for all of their medical needs: doctor visits, special studies, and hospitalization; the HMO employs doctors (primary ones and specialists), usually on a full-time basis and contract with, or own hospitals; the theory behind this program is that the number of studies requested and hospital-use are under the control of physicians, and therefore the fewer tests done, and the less hospitalization recommended, increases the pool of fees available to be divided among the member physicians; also, the fewer surgical and other specialty consultations obtained, the greater the income of the primary physician (first-to-see-patient) members of the plan; HMOs can be non-profit (except for its physicians) or for-profit organizations who employ the physicians - by, 1992 an estimated 2/3 of HMOs were investor owned (for varieties of HMOs, see Chapter 1).

Healthy revenues: see sin taxes.

Implicit rationing: decisions as to who gets care, or which part of medical care, not being legally mandated but, nevertheless, induced by the nature of the delivery system; implicit rationing is generally micro-rationing that is done without open discussion, and therefore not "visible" to the public.

Incremental changes: alterations of a medical-care system to counter unwanted consequences, rather than reform its basic characteristics or ideology; generally refers to changes made for purposes of cost-containment.

Individual practice association (IPA): individual practice associations are a form of HMO consisting of a group of physicians who maintain their own offices and care for subscribers to a prepaid plan at a reduced rate fee-for-service basis (also referred to as a "network-type HMO").

Jackson Hole Group: a group of economists, politicians, insurance executives, providers and others interested in medical-care financing and planning that meets in Jackson Hole, Wyoming, chaired by Alain Enthoven and Paul Ellwood (originator of concept of managed competition);, group endorses Enthoven's program for reforming the U.S. medical-care system, referred to as the Jackson Hole Initiative (Chapter V-2A).

Job-lock: when a worker cannot change jobs for fear of losing health insurance coverage.

Lock-In: a feature of a program (usually Medicaid) which restricts choice of a provider by a beneficiary who has over-used services.

Lock-Out: a feature of a program (usually Medicaid) which limits the participation of so-called "over-zealous" providers.

Long-term care services (LTC): health, social, housing, transportation,and other supportive services needed by persons with physical, mental or cognitive limitations sufficient to compromise independent living (a large percentage of which are the aged).

Macro-rationing (of medical care): is when a government limits the total funds allocated to medical care; a mechanism that restricts the amounts allocated to medical care, such as using a "single payer" to negotiate with providers; to be contrasted with micro-rationing.

Managed care: Managed care takes three forms. In the first, physicians in a group, or staff-type, HMO have an economic incentive to curtail, so-called, unnecessary care; In the second, patients either are assigned to, or choose, a primary physician from a panel recruited by insurers into an HMO, PPO or PPI and who supervise their care; with this type of managed care, insurance companies (or any other payer) has the power, by denying reimbursement, to force physicians to conform to their rules against "wasteful and unnecessary practices"; in managed care, doctors not only receive reduced fees but also all studies and treatments must initiate with, or be approved by, the managing doctor; A third form of managed care takes place when insurers insist on their reviewing each case (by nurses or doctors they employ) before agreeing to pay for designated diagnostic studies or treatments.

Managed competition (Enthoven or Jackson Hole Plan): When entities such as large employers or a government agency, who have enough resources to be knowledgeable and represent sufficiently large numbers of potential patients to be a potent force, are required or given incentive (like being able to deduct only the cost of the least expensive approved plan from corporate taxes) to do the negotiating with providers of medical care as to costs, including services and quality of services, and not leaving choice to uninformed, or unmotivated, or weak individuals (or companies). This is done to overcome the usual blunting of the medical-care market by personal considerations and make it more like other commodity markets. Providers are forced to join together in groups to compete for patients on the basis of being less costly, and the quantity and quality of the services they offer. All this should lower costs of medical care by increasing competition among providers.

Means test: requires a person to disclose assets to prove economic necessity and therefore eligible to be a beneficiary of a govern mental program.

Medicaid: a health insurance program for the poor, funded 50% to 70% by the federal government and partly by the individual states; it is administered by the states.

Medical care: an aspect of health care that is concerned with the diagnosis and treatment of disease after it has developed; see health care.

Medicare: a health insurance program for people 65 and older and some people under 65 who are disabled or have end-stage kidney disease; it is funded by the federal government and managed by the Health Care Financing Agency (HCFA); it has two parts: Part A pays for hospital care and Part B for doctors' services and outpatient hospital services.

Medicare volume performance standard (MVPS): volume performance standard applied to Medicare.

Medigap insurance: An insurance policy paid for by a beneficiary of Medicare, to cover medical-care charges not reimbursed by Medicare - such as deductibles and copayments required by Medicare regulations; same as gap insurance.

Micro-rationing of medical care: decisions made about which individuals shall have access to a specific procedure, the supply of which is most often limited by the total of funds available, or budgeted (macro-rationed), for medical care; may be implicit or explicit rationing.

National health insurance (NHI): a publicly financed (via taxes) insurance program to cover the entire population, such as the Canadian system; to be contrasted with Universal Health insurance.

Necessary care: medical care that prolongs life or improves its quality.

Network-type HMO: see "individual practice association (IPA)" and primary care network.

Outcomes and appropriateness-of-services research (or studies): research into the final results of a treatments' effect on a patients' illnesses or complaints, from which conclusions can be drawn as to the appropriateness (or rightness) of the use of particular treatments in an individual patient (while a treatment may be of value overall, it could be ineffective in a specific individual situation); in some instances outcomes research also implies studying the cost-effectiveness of treatments; these studies are suggested as a way to eliminate ineffective treatments and thus help contain medical-care costs.

Out-of-pocket: Refers to monies paid by patients, and not reimbursable from insurers (third parties).

Partial Payment of Premium: When an employer or the government provides insurance for individuals, requiring the insured to pay part of the premium ("partial payment"); it is helpful in guiding individuals choosing plans that provides services with the lowest premiums.

Patient Outcomes Research Team Program (PORTs): Multidisciplinary teams set up by the U.S. government through the Department of Health Agency for Health Care Policy and Research to evaluate the results (outcomes) of treatment of specific disease items. Initial funding, in 1992, was for $40 million.

Peer review: A method of containing costs by having physicians review the practices of other physicians. See: Professional Standards Review Organizations; Second Opinion Programs.

Physician profiling: analysis of a physician's practice pattern, including use of diagnostic procedures, referrals (both to hospitals and other physicians) and, especially, drug prescribing trend.

Play-or-Pay Program: A proposal to supply medical insurance cover age to those previously uninsured by mandating that employers supply health insurance to all of their employees (play), or pay a percentage of their payroll to a public agency which, in turn, supplies the insurance coverage to the employee.

Point-of-service-plan: a managed-care plan (HMO, PPO or primary care network) that allows patients to use providers outside the network, but demands a higher copayment for doing so.

Poverty Level: in the United States in 1992 it was $14,343 for a family of four and $7141 for an individual.

Pre-admission and/or pre-procedure certification: before doing a procedure on, or hospitalizing a patient, the physician must obtain the permission of the third-party payer, or else the latter will not reimburse the patient for the cost.

Pre-procedure certification: see entry immediately above.

Preferred Provider Insurance (PPI): Health insurance that only provides for services from a preferred-provider-organization (PPO).

Preferred Provider Organizations (PPOs): are groups of hospitals and/or physicians offering care on a fee-for-service basis but at reduced rates in return for a guaranteed volume of patients.

Primary Care: medical care provided by the first physician to be consulted by a patient, usually presumed to be unreferred from another physician (a general practitioner in all countries abroad and, in United States, a general internist, an obstetrician or a general pediatrician as well). Sometimes called "ambulatory care".

Primary care network: or "case-managed care" places primary care physicians practicing in their own offices at some economic risk in an effort to make them more prudent users of medical resources for their patients; primary care network are augmented by a panel of specialists and all referrals to them must be approved by the primary physician; primary care network physicians are paid on a per capita basis and if excessive costs are incurred by their patients their incomes are, or could be, reduced; these are a form of "managed care" and analogous to an HMO.

Primary Care Physicians: physicians first visited by patients (see "primary care", above).

Professional Standards Review Organizations (PSROs): A form of peer review with the objective of containing expenditures by Medicare and Medicaid, but often used by private insurers. Admissions and lengths of stay in hospitals are reviewed by committees of their own staff physicians and the standards applied in this review are established by local (city, county, or similar areas) organizations.

Prospective payment system (PPS): A method to reimburse providers prospectively. Conceived to replace the cost-plus method of reimbursement, and specifically legislated to apply to hospital Medicare payments via the diagnostic-related-groups (DRGs) method.

Provider: a provider (in medical care) is a physician, hospital, HMO, pharmacy, laboratory, etc. that provides services or supplies to a patient or patients.

Purchaser: is a patient that pays for the services of a provider; or an entity, such as an insurer or a plan, that pays (or reimburses) a provider on behalf of a patient.

Queuing: in medical care is to having to wait, in line, for a service; it is a form of micro-rationing, more or less explicit, and occurs in those countries where the global budgeting of medical-care resources limits its availability.

Refundable tax credits: when tax credits exceeds the family's tax liability, the difference is remitted by the government to them in cash; see "tax credit".

Resource based relative value scale for physician reimbursement (RBRVSs): a method for calculating physicians' fees based on the relative values that have been established for its three components: 1) a work component that reflects physicians time and in tensity; 2) a practice expense component that reflects overhead; 3) a malpractice component reflecting malpractice costs.

Risk avoidance: term used to describe procedure of insurers when they avoid insuring individuals deemed to be very prone, for one or another reason, to use medical care.

Risk-rated insurance premium: see casualty-rated premiums.

Rule-of-rescue: No matter what guidelines are set up, if a treatment is known to exist, it will be obtained for an individual.

Second opinion program: This is a peer review program specifically designed to reduce the amount of elective surgery done. It re quires that before an elective operation is done and the patient is reimbursed for its costs, that another surgeon agree on the necessity, or at least the desirability, that it be done.

Self-referral: denotes when a physician refers a patient to a facility for diagnosis or treatment in which the physician has a monetary interest. The inference is that in such a circumstance the physician will over-utilize the facility by recommending unnecessary care.

Single-payer system: a macro-rationing, cost-containment measure in which payment for services comes from one source, usually a governmental agency or a government-sponsored consortium of insurers. It prevents providers from playing off one payer against another, and saves by administrative simplification.

Sin taxes: Taxes on tobacco or alcohol (substances that are legal, but harmful to one's health); also called healthy revenues.

Spend-down-assets: means depleting oneself of assets to qualify for long-term care by Medicaid. Usually refers to elderly with some assets, but insufficient to cover the continued long-term care they require.

State-mandated-special-benefits laws: are those that require insurance companies to make payment for special services (as treatment for drug and alcohol abuse, chiropractic care, in vitro fertilization, acupuncture, wigs, etc.). Seven hundred such state laws are on the books and are said to raise insurance rates by as much as 20%.

Tax credit: is an amount subtracted from the total of income taxes owed, "dollar for dollar"; see "refundable tax credits".

Tax deduction: is an amount subtracted from a tax-payer's total income in computing their taxable income; the actual saving to tax-payers is equal to the amount deductible, multiplied by their tax rate (at most, in 1992, 31%).

Tertiary Care: The ultimate in specialty medical care; usually assumed to be provided in large medical centers (often, but not necessarily, teaching hospitals) with referral of patients from primary physicians and other specialists.

Third-Party payer: An entity (usually an insurance company or a government program) that pays providers for services rendered patients.

Tiered care: varying levels of amount and quality of medical care; usually implying that the level of quality and/or amount of care is related to the patient's ability to pay for it; frequently referred to as "two-tiered" care.

Unbundle: billing separately for components of an integral service (to obtain higher reimbursement than a provider would obtain from one all-encompassing bill).

Unbundling of services: Unbundling is when services previously supplied by a hospital, such as x-rays or anesthesia, are separated out and billed by ostensibly independent physicians and paid by Part B of Medicare (physician reimbursement) rather than included in Part A payment (for hospital care). Also a means of circumventing DRG payments.

Uncompensated care: Medical care for which the provider is not re-imbursed, usually provided to patients who are uninsured, and the costs of which almost always are "shifted" (cost-shifting), to be paid for through increase in the premiums of those with private insurance or in taxes supporting government programs as Medicare and Medicaid.

Universal health insurance (UHI): any insurance system decreed for covering the entire population but supported by a mixture of public and private funds, as in Germany or the Netherlands; to be contrasted with national health insurance.

Unnecessary care: medical care that neither preserves life nor enhances its quality; usually refers to practices of physicians merely to amplify their incomes or for defense against malpractice suits (defensive medicine).

Value-added-tax (VAT): a tax added to the price of a product, calculated as a percentage of its value and payable by the consumer; most often such a tax is imposed on an item at every stage of its production and the total tax is reflected in the final price to the consumer; mentioned in some programs as a means of financing reforms.

Vertical integration: is a coordinated system of physician and hospital services set up to contract to deliver medical care: as staff model HMOs that employ physicians and own hospitals; physician group practices that own hospitals, HMOs or PPOs; physicians and hospitals form a joint venture; IPAs that join or own hospitals; hospitals that employ physicians, operate HMOs or IPAs, own nursing homes, etc.

Volume performance standards: are expenditure targets set for physicians' services to make sure they do not increase the number or intensity of services to compensate for any curtailment of their fees under RBRVSs; if targets are exceeded, the yearly adjustment rate for physicians' fees would be reduced, but if actual expenditures on fees for physicians is below target, the adjustment rate could be increased.

ACRONYMS

AARP	American Association of Retired People
AMA	American Medical Association
CHAMPUS	Civilian Health And Medical Programs of the Uniformed Services
CMO	Competitive Medical Organization
COLA	Cost-Of-Living Adjustment
CON	Certificate Of Need
CPI	Consumer Price Index
DRG	Diagnostic Related Group
EHI	Employee Health Insurance law
ERISA	Employee Retirement Income Security Act
GP	General Practitioner
GDP	Gross Domestic Product
GNP	Gross National Product
HCFA	Health Care Financing Agency
HIA	Health Insurance Association of America
HIPC	Health Insurance Purchasing Cooperative
HHS	U.S. Department of Health and Human Services
HMO	Health Maintenance Organization
IPA	Independent Practice Association
LTC	Long-Term Care
MVPS	Medical Volume Performance Standard
NHI	National Health Insurance
NHP	National Health Program
NHS	National Health Service (British)
OECD	Organization for Economic Cooperation and Development
PORTs	Patient Outcomes Research Team Programs
PPI	Preferred Provider Insurance
PPO	Preferred Provider Organization
PRO	Professional Review Organization
PPS	Prospective payment System
PSRO	Professional Standards Review Organization
RBRVS	Resource Based Relative Value Scale
UHI	Universal Health Insurance
VAT	Value Added Tax

INDEX

152

ADDENDA

September 15, 1993

Early in September 1993, the Clinton Administration unofficially released their program to reform the medical-care system—planning to officially present it to Congress at the end of that month. Their program is essentially that of the Jackson Hole Group for managed-competition and managed-care. However, fearing managed-competition won't be sufficiently effective in containing costs, the Clinton program adds a mechanism for imposing caps on insurance premiums. And, if necessary, it will also place caps on fees to providers. The caps are to be set by a National Health Board in line with what it determines should be the global budget for medical care.

Another board will determine the quality of medical care being delivered by the various medical-care plans and by doctors and hospitals. This will assist consumers in making choices. The board will also monitor the creation of a health security card for every American and a standard reimbursement form so as to reduce administrative expenses and hassles with paperwork.

To insure the uninsured, it has been estimated that $50 to $80 billion is required annually for at least a few years until savings from competition accumulate. Rather than using taxes to cover these costs, the Administration intends to phase in their program gradually and raise the tax on tobacco. This is estimated to yield $10 billion annually and would be popular. Further savings are intended by reducing the annual rate of the growth of Medicare by 65% (estimated to yield $18 billion annually) and cutting the annual growth of Medicaid by 75%.

The Administration's struggles in these last months have centered on two points—as will, undoubtedly, future discussions. First, how to finance coverage of all the previously uninsured without onerous taxation, and second, what to include in a basic plan that must hold down costs and yet satisfy the Administration's own agenda while increasing the appeal of their program.

The Administration has aggravated its cost-containment problem by including the following benefits in its basic health plan: mental-health care—demanded by some to be covered equally with physical ailments despite its indeterminate results and open-ended costs; costs of drugs and long-term care to assuage the outspoken elderly; preventive care items, which are popular but some of which could cost more than they would save; and a beginning on coverage for dental care. All these benefits could require an extra $100 billion annually.

The Administration's dilemma arises from three basic contradictions:

1. Repairing one of the two major issues creating the crisis—the large numbers of uninsured people—obviously aggravates the other important issue—restraining the escalating costs of medical care.

2. These same two issues evoke opposing facets of human nature—the altruistic instinct upon which we base our moral code and which dictates that medical care is a right of all individuals, and the egoistic instinct (or self-interest) which doesn't want to pay for altruism's demands. This second contradiction pits moral ideology against political reality.

3. The third contradiction arises from the Administration's belief that cost-containment eventually requires global budgeting with caps on spending—macro-rationing procedures that inevitably lead to micro-rationing. But even the very hint of rationing is unacceptable to the electorate.

By mid-September 1993, criticism of the Clinton program focused on the following points:

1. It was too expensive for small businesses and would force many to close;

2. Caps on spending and fees would eventually destroy the very competition that supporters of managed-competition rely upon to contain costs;

3. Creation of state sponsors—some suggest there should be as many as two hundred or more—and the various national boards with supporting staffs would increase government bureaucracy and add as much as $2 billion annually to administrative costs.

4. Finally, some criticize the Clinton program because imposing caps would impose rationing for individuals, as do all nations

that use the macro-rationing single-payer and global budgeting techniques to control costs.

Despite the often-repeated forecast of a monumental struggle in Congress over medical-care reform, initial criticism of the Clinton medical-care reform initiative seemed muted. Perhaps the country is so anxious for reform that opposition to the Administration's program—even though it promised to revolutionize the delivery of medical care in the U.S.—may prove less strident and prolonged than anticipated. The serious and lengthy struggle may occur after enactment, however, depending on how well the reforms succeed in attaining their objectives and satisfying the electorate.